I NEED TO GO TO THE

TOILET

A CARER'S GUIDE TO CATHETER CARE:

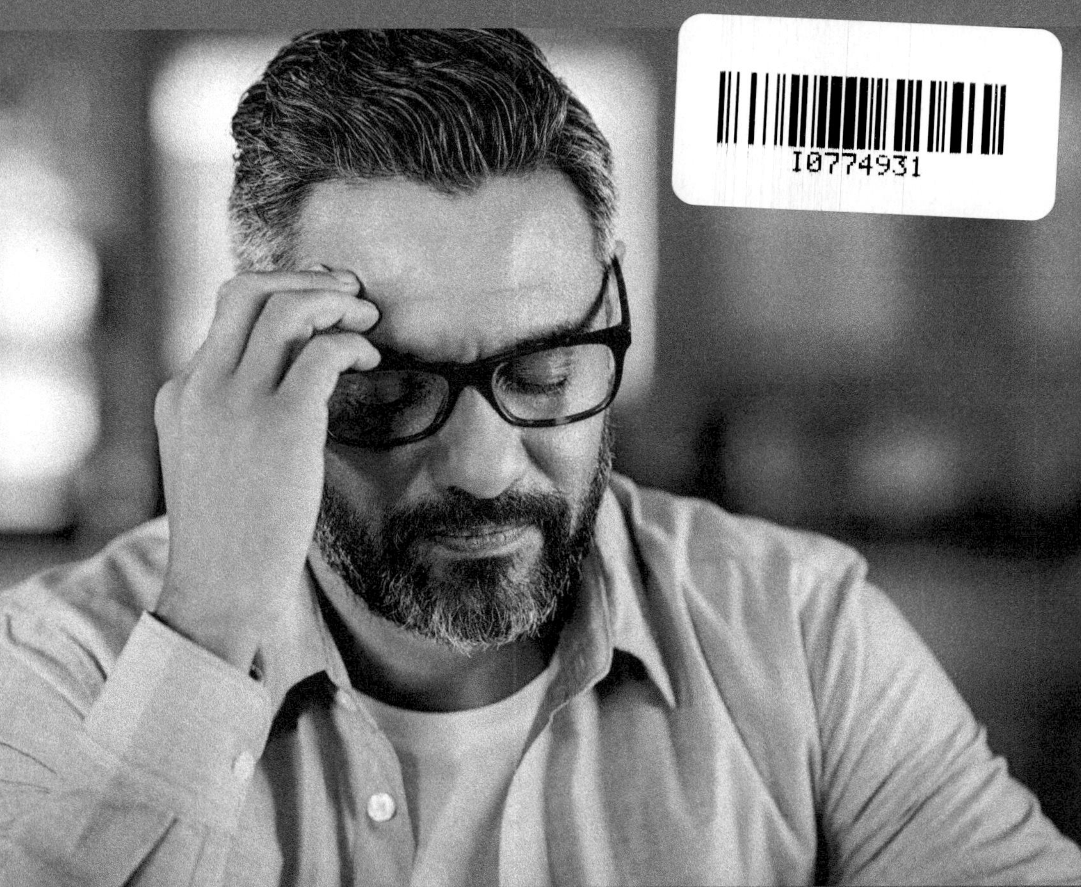

ROY LANGSTAFFE

BY THE SAME AUTHOR

A Different Kind of Normal: A Carer's Guide To Autism and How To Support

Me, Myself and THE OTHER ONE: A Carers Guide To Mental Health and What To Expect in Care

The I Series:

I Need To Go To The Toilet: A Carers Guide To Catheter Care

I Can Be A Handful: A Carers Guide To Male Personal Care

With Angela Langstaffe

I am A Lady You Know: A Carers Guide to Female Personal Care

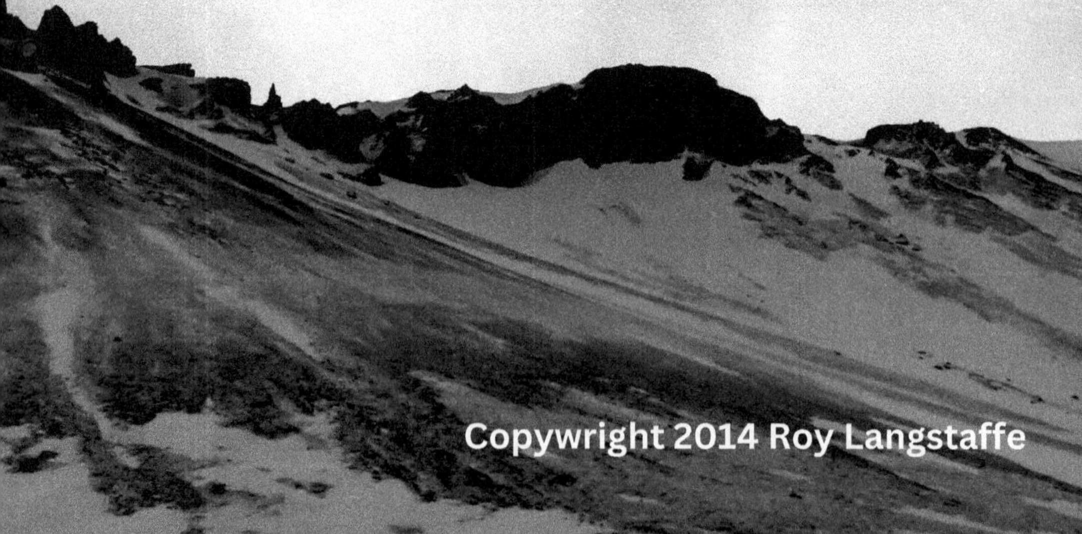

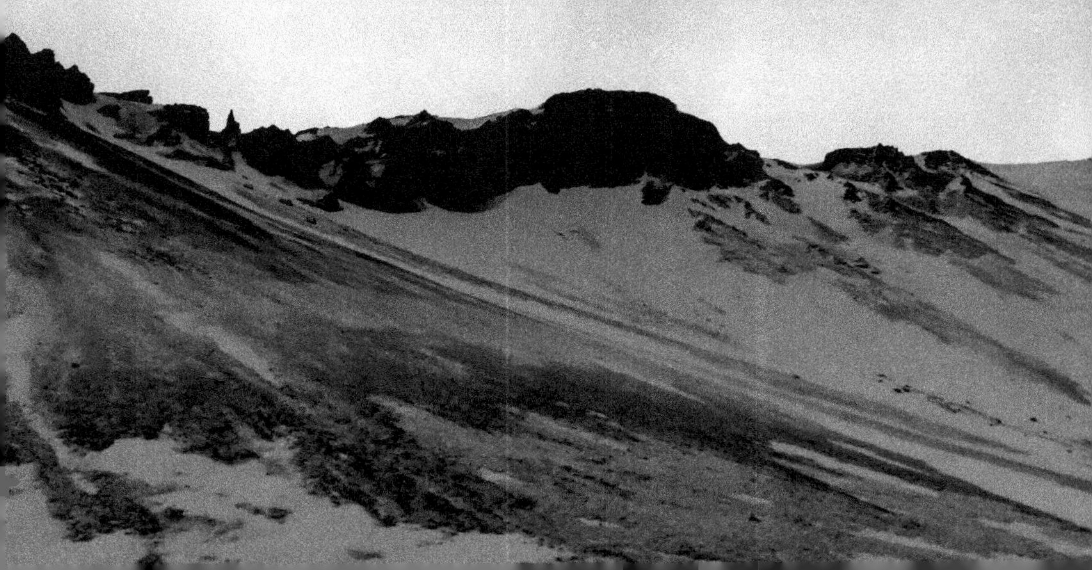

This book is dedicated to all those amazing carers out there that really make a difference.

I Need To Go To The Toilet

A CARER'S GUIDE TO CATHETER CARE:

Hello, I'm Roy Langstaffe, a seasoned trainer and coach with a deep passion for caregiving. With years of experience, I excel in guiding individuals to become exceptional caregivers.

I collaborate with diverse organizations to elevate caregiving standards and practices. Beyond my training endeavors, I'm also an author and aspiring musician, showcasing my multifaceted approach to life.

My commitment to the well-being of caregivers is evident in my tireless advocacy and dedication. With compassion and creativity at the forefront, I strive to make a meaningful impact on the lives of caregivers and those they care for, ensuring their sanity and strength are upheld.

I hope you enjoy this e book and find some knowledge that helps you!

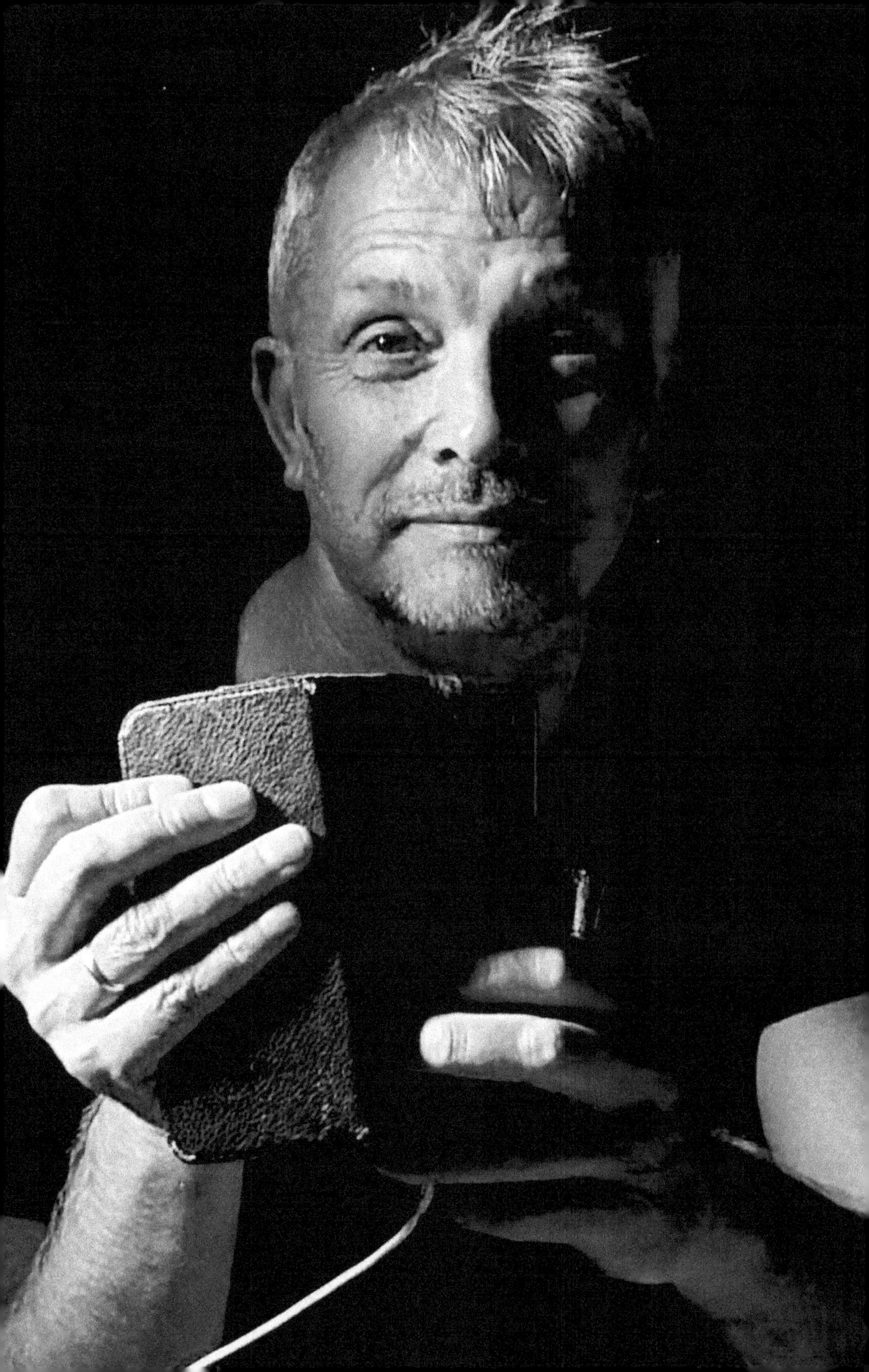

CHAPTER 1
INTRODUCTION

What is Catheterisation?

Welcome to Chapter 1 of "A Carer's Guide to Catheter Care – I Need to Go to the Toilet." In this chapter, we'll embark on a journey to demystify the world of catheterisation—a vital topic that, while serious, can be approached with a touch of wit to make the learning process engaging and memorable. So, let's dive into the essentials of catheterisation and understand its role in healthcare.

What is Catheterisation?

Imagine your bladder is like a water balloon that occasionally needs to be emptied. Sometimes, due to various health conditions, it needs a little help to do its job. That's where catheterization comes in. Simply put, catheterisation is the process of inserting a thin, flexible tube—known as a catheter—into the bladder to drain urine. It's a procedure that, despite its straightforward purpose, plays a crucial role in modern healthcare.

The purpose of catheterisation extends beyond just draining urine. It can also be used to collect sterile urine samples, deliver medications directly into the bladder, and maintain bladder drainage during and after surgeries. Think of it as the Swiss Army knife of medical procedures: versatile, dependable, and essential in many situations.

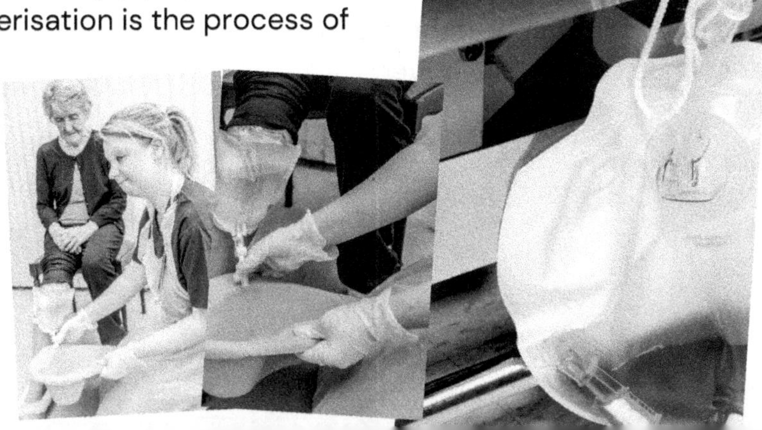

The Purpose of Catheterisation

1. **Urinary Drainage**: The primary purpose of catheterisation is to relieve urinary retention. Whether due to an obstruction, nerve-related issues, or post-surgery, a catheter ensures that urine doesn't hang around longer than it should. Without proper drainage, the urinary system could face serious complications, including infections and kidney damage.
2. **Diagnostic Procedures:** Catheterisation allows healthcare providers to collect sterile urine samples directly from the bladder, ensuring that no external contaminants interfere with diagnostic tests. It's like getting a backstage pass to see what's really going on in the urinary tract.
3. **Surgical Use:** During and after certain surgeries, keeping the bladder empty is essential. A catheter helps manage this, reducing the risk of complications and allowing the surgical team to focus on the task at hand.
4. **Medication Administration**: Sometimes, medications need to go directly to the source. Catheters can deliver drugs straight into the bladder, ensuring targeted treatment for conditions like interstitial cystitis or bladder cancer.
5. **Hydration and Nutrition:** In cases where oral intake isn't possible, catheters can also be used to administer fluids and nutrients. This is particularly important in critically ill patients who need every ounce of care to recover.

How Do Catheters Work?

The concept of a catheter is deceptively simple: it's just a tube, right? Well, yes and no. While the basic idea is straightforward, the design and functionality of catheters are quite sophisticated. Let's break it down:

1. **Materials**: Catheters are typically made from medical-grade materials like silicone, latex, or polyurethane. Each material has its own advantages. For instance, silicone is flexible and less likely to cause allergic reactions, while latex is more pliable and can be more comfortable for short-term use.
2. **Design**: The design of a catheter varies depending on its intended use. Some catheters are straight and rigid, while others are more flexible. Indwelling catheters (those meant to stay in place for a while) often have a balloon at the end. Once inserted, the balloon is inflated to keep the catheter securely in the bladder.
3. **Insertion**: Catheters can be inserted through the urethra or, in some cases, directly into the bladder through a small incision in the abdomen (suprapubic catheterization). The method of insertion depends on the patient's needs and the healthcare provider's assessment.
4. **Drainage:** Once in place, the catheter allows urine to flow from the bladder into a collection bag. This can be done continuously (as with indwelling catheters) or intermittently (as with straight or intermittent catheters).
5. **Removal:** The removal process is straightforward. For indwelling catheters, the balloon is deflated, and the catheter is gently pulled out. Intermittent catheters are removed immediately after the bladder is emptied.

The Role of Catheters in Healthcare

Catheters are unsung heroes in the medical world. They may not have the glamour of cutting-edge surgical robots or the intrigue of new pharmaceutical breakthroughs, but their role is indispensable. Here's a glimpse into their significance:

1. **Hospital Care:** In hospital settings, catheters are used to manage patients who are unable to control their bladder function due to illness, injury, or surgery. They help maintain hygiene and prevent complications, making the patient's stay more comfortable and safer.
2. **Home Care:** For many patients, catheterization is part of their daily routine at home. Whether due to chronic conditions like spinal cord injuries or temporary needs post-surgery, catheters enable these individuals to lead more independent lives.
3. **Elderly Care**: In long-term care facilities, catheters are often used to manage urinary incontinence in elderly patients. This not only helps in maintaining hygiene but also preserves the dignity of residents, allowing them to enjoy a better quality of life.
4. **Specialized Treatments**: In urology, catheters are vital for certain diagnostic tests and treatments. They provide direct access to the bladder, facilitating procedures that would otherwise be difficult or impossible to perform.
5. **Emergency Situations**: In emergency medicine, catheters can be lifesavers. For patients with acute urinary retention or severe injuries, timely catheterization can prevent serious complications and stabilize their condition.

Appreciating the Unsung Hero

Now, let's add a dash of humour to lighten the mood. Imagine if catheters could talk—what stories they would tell! They'd probably regale us with tales of heroism, from saving patients in emergency rooms to helping the elderly enjoy a good night's sleep without the worry of accidents. They'd boast about their flexibility, adaptability, and crucial role in the grand theatre of healthcare.

Think of a catheter as a dedicated postal worker, tirelessly delivering "liquid mail" from the bladder to the collection bag, rain or shine, day or night. Or picture it as a reliable butler, discreetly managing the household's less glamorous tasks with utmost efficiency and grace. Without these unassuming heroes, the smooth functioning of many medical procedures and patient care routines would be much more challenging.

Conclusion

Catheterisation might not be the most glamorous topic in healthcare, but its importance cannot be overstated. Understanding what catheterisation is, its purposes, and how catheters work provides a solid foundation for carers and healthcare providers alike. With this knowledge, you are better equipped to provide compassionate, effective care that preserves the dignity and comfort of those who rely on catheterisation.

So, as we continue our journey through "A Carer's Guide to Catheter Care – I Need to Go to the Toilet," remember to appreciate the humble catheter—not just as a medical device, but as a vital tool that makes a significant difference in the lives of many. And who knows? You might just find yourself chuckling at the thought of a catheter with a personality, ready to share its adventures from the front lines of patient care.

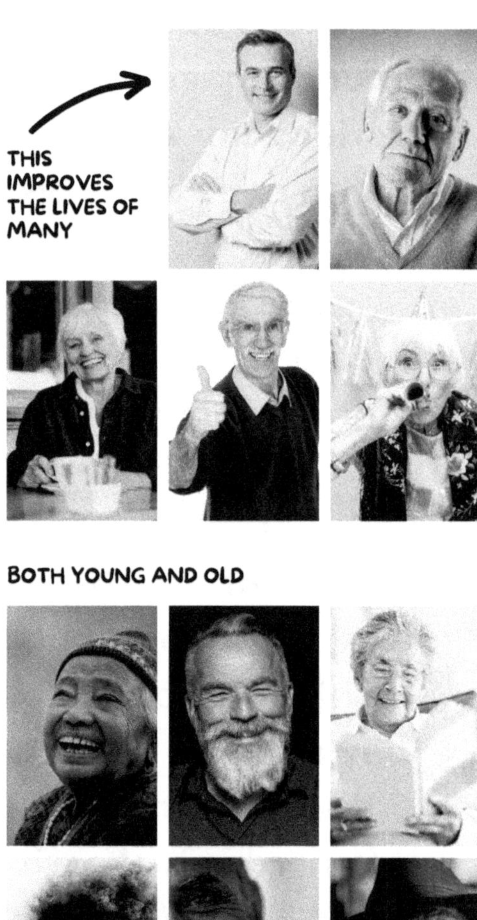

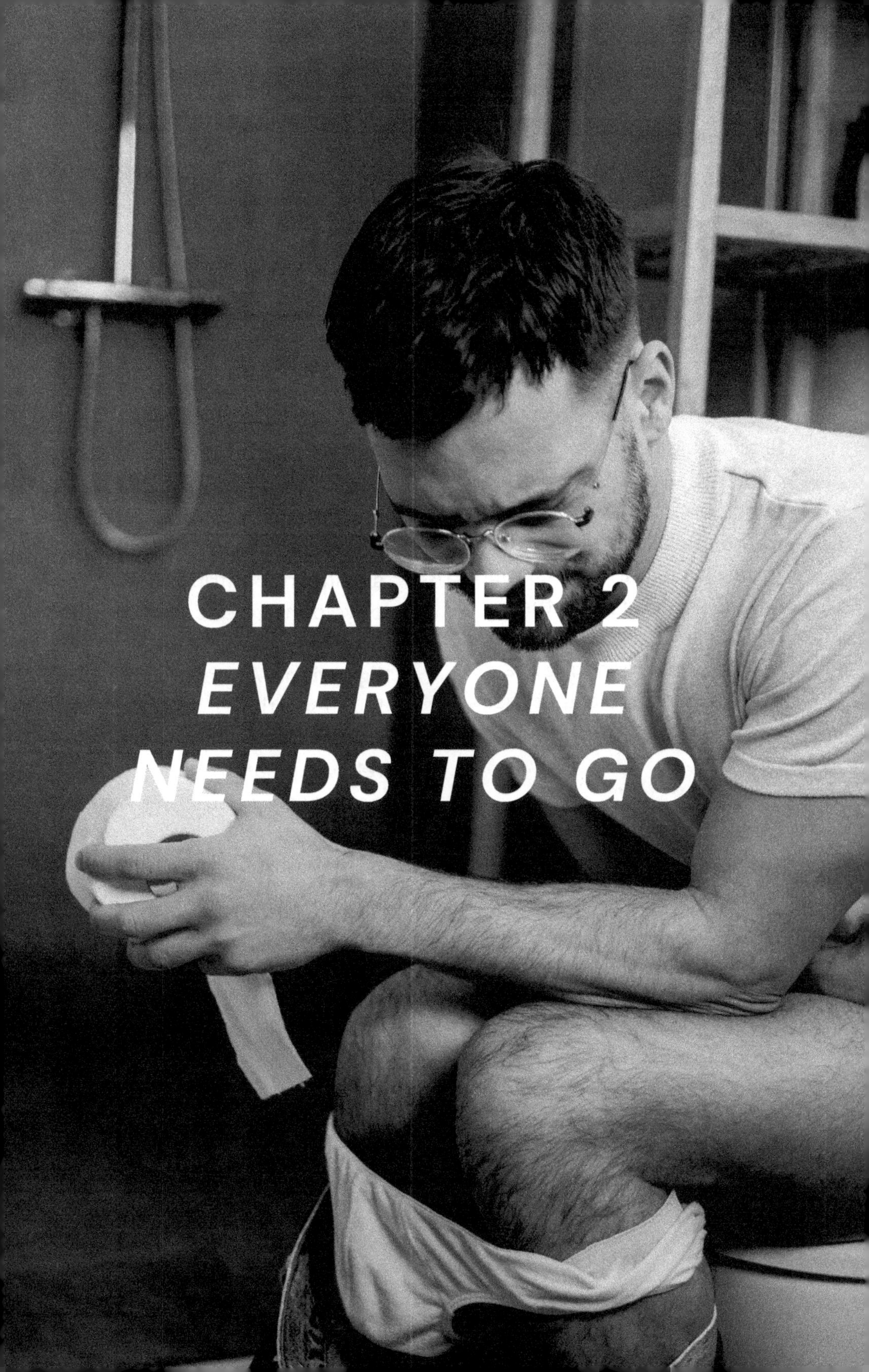

CHAPTER 2
EVERYONE
NEEDS TO GO

A Brief History of Catheterisation

In this chapter, we delve into the fascinating history of catheterisation, tracing its evolution from ancient techniques to the modern marvels we rely on today. It's a journey that highlights human ingenuity and the relentless quest to improve medical care, ensuring that everyone, regardless of their condition, can "go" with dignity and ease.

Evolution of Catheterisation

Techniques and Materials Catheterisation, the process of inserting a tube into the body to drain or deliver fluids, is an ancient practice. Its history spans thousands of years, reflecting the evolving understanding of human anatomy and the relentless pursuit of more effective medical treatments.

Ancient Beginnings

The earliest records of catheter use date back to ancient civilizations. The Egyptians, Greeks, and Romans all made significant contributions to the development of catheterization.

Egyptians: As early as 3000 BCE, Egyptian physicians used hollow reeds and metals to relieve urinary retention. These rudimentary catheters were simple yet effective, demonstrating early medical practitioners' ingenuity.

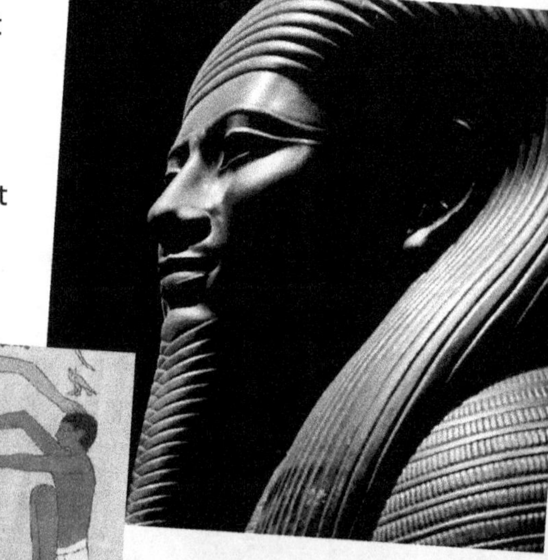

Greeks: Hippocrates, the father of medicine, mentioned the use of metal tubes to treat urinary obstructions in the 5th century BCE. The Greeks were among the first to document medical procedures systematically, paving the way for future advancements.

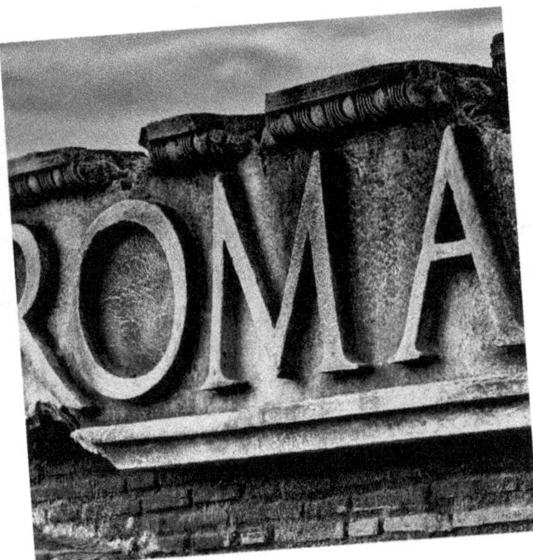

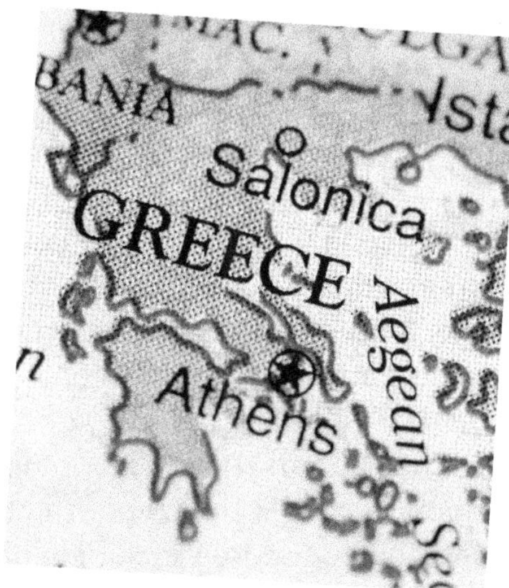

Romans: In ancient Rome, catheters made from lead or bronze were commonly used. Soranus of Ephesus, a prominent Roman physician, described catheterisation techniques in his medical texts around the 1st century CE. These early devices were rigid and uncomfortable but provided critical relief for those suffering from urinary retention.

Medieval Innovations

During the medieval period, the knowledge and use of catheters spread across Europe and the Middle East. Islamic scholars like Avicenna and Al-Zahrawi (Abulcasis) advanced medical science, including catheterisation techniques.

Renaissance and Early Modern Period

The Renaissance era brought renewed interest in science and medicine. Anatomical knowledge expanded, leading to more sophisticated medical instruments, including catheters.

19th Century Breakthroughs

The 19th century was a period of rapid medical advancement, including significant improvements in catheter technology.

Antoine-Joseph Jobert de Lamballe: In the early 1800s, French surgeon Jobert de Lamballe introduced the use of rubber in catheter manufacturing. Rubber catheters were more flexible and less likely to cause trauma to the urethra.

Thomas Lister: The development of antiseptic techniques by Thomas Lister in the mid-19th century revolutionized surgery and medical procedures, including catheterisation. Sterilization reduced the risk of infection, making catheter use safer for patients.

Foley Catheter: Perhaps the most significant breakthrough came in 1935 when American urologist Dr. Frederic Foley invented the Foley catheter. This indwelling catheter featured a balloon at the tip that could be inflated to keep the catheter in place within the bladder. The Foley catheter remains a cornerstone of modern catheterisation, widely used in hospitals and care settings worldwide.

Milestones in the Development of Modern Catheter Care
As we move into the 20th and 21st centuries, the evolution of catheter care has continued at a remarkable pace. Innovations in materials, design, and techniques have transformed catheterisation into a safer, more effective, and more comfortable procedure for patients.

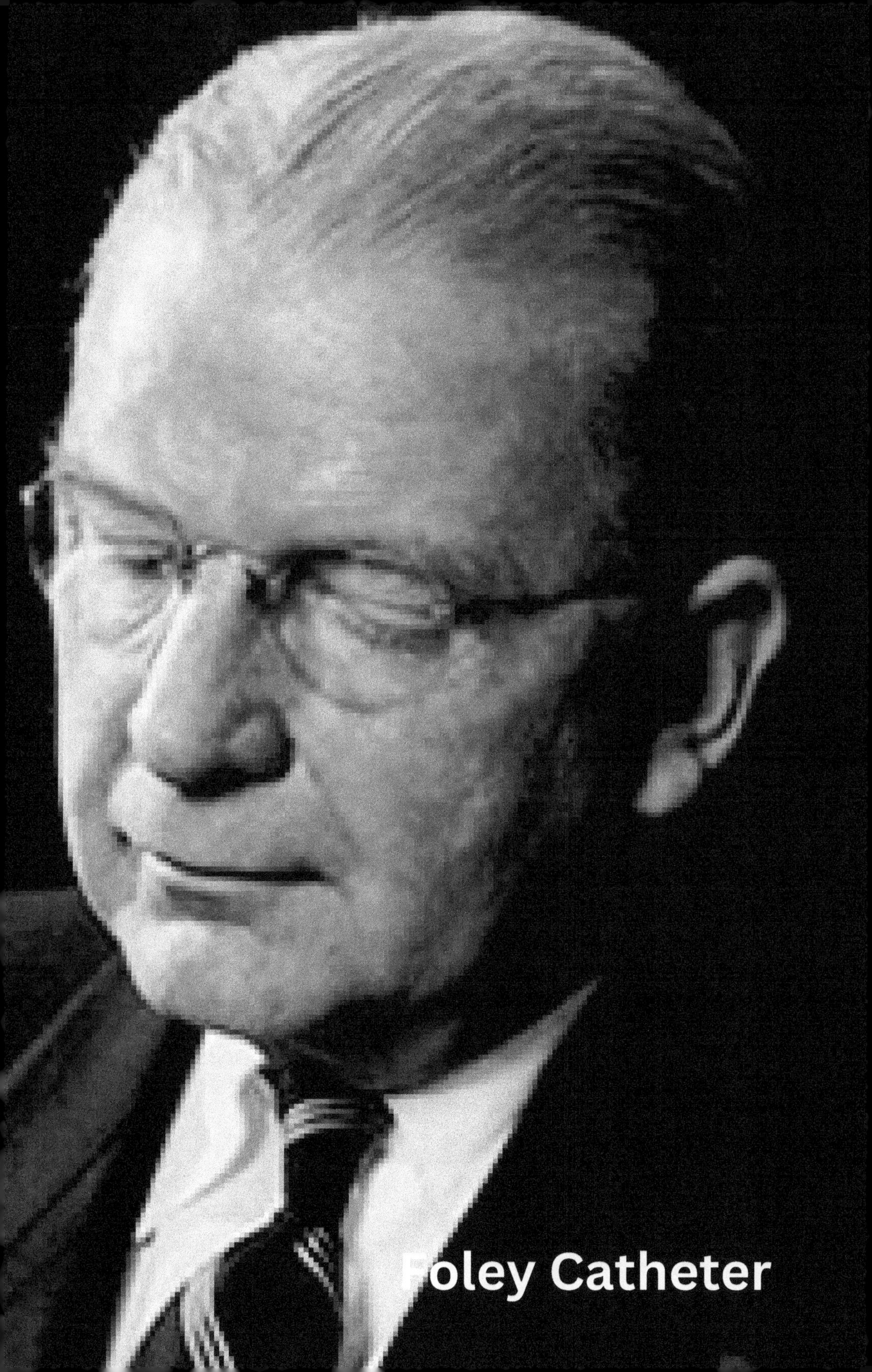
Foley Catheter

Advances In Materials

Modern catheters are made from a variety of advanced materials, each chosen for specific properties that enhance patient comfort and safety.

Silicone: Silicone catheters are biocompatible, flexible, and less likely to cause allergic reactions. They can be used for long-term catheterisation due to their durability and low risk of causing irritation.

Polyurethane: Polyurethane catheters are strong and flexible, making them ideal for both short-term and long-term use. They are also resistant to kinking, ensuring reliable drainage.

Hydrophilic Coatings: Many modern catheters feature hydrophilic coatings that become slippery when wet, reducing friction and making insertion more comfortable for the patient.

Innovations in Design
The design of catheters has also evolved to meet the diverse needs of patients and healthcare providers. We will explore more in the later chapters.

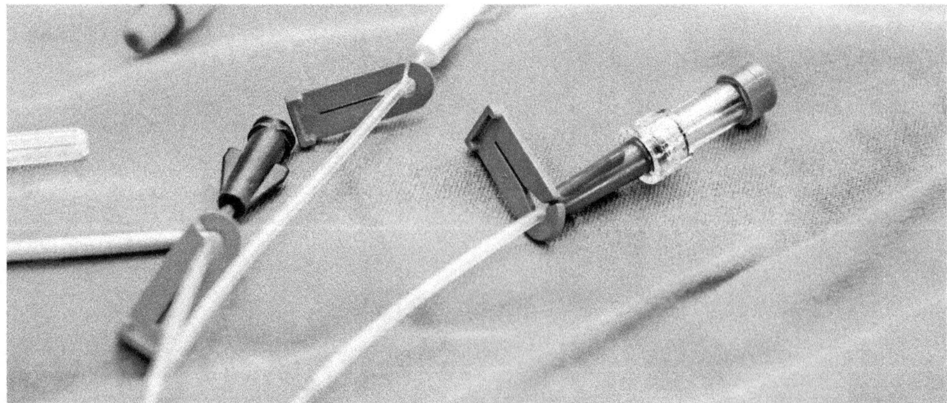

Conclusion

The history of catheterisation is a testament to human innovation and the relentless pursuit of better healthcare solutions. From the rudimentary hollow reeds of ancient Egypt to the sophisticated, high-tech catheters of today, each advancement has brought us closer to providing patients with safe, effective, and dignified care.

Understanding this history not only gives us an appreciation for the progress that has been made but also highlights the importance of ongoing innovation and education in catheter care.

As carers and healthcare providers, it is our responsibility to stay informed about the latest developments, ensuring that we can offer the best possible care to those who need it.

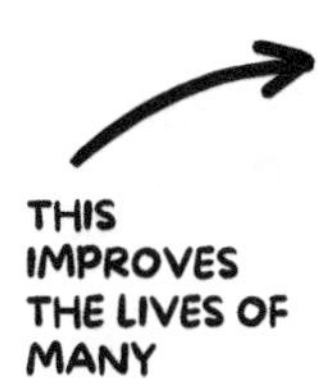

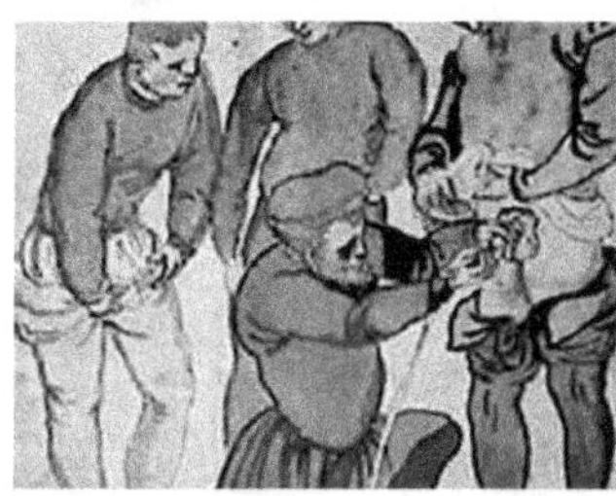

MEDICAL ADVANCES THROUGH THE AGES

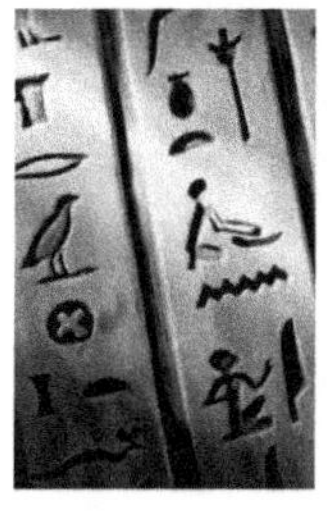
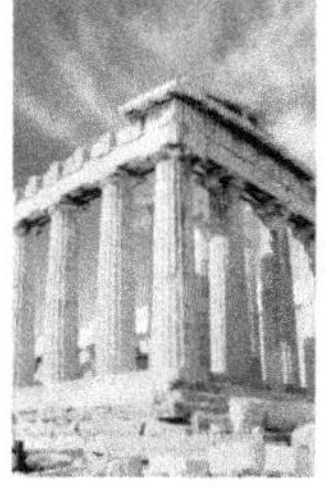
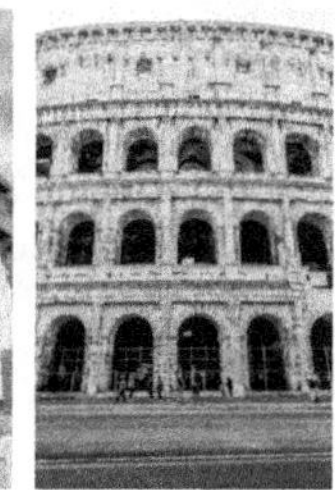
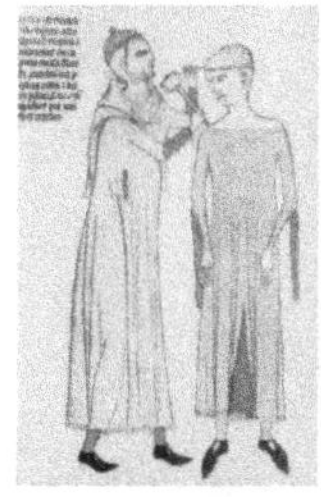
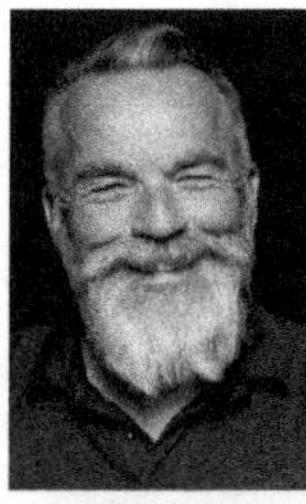
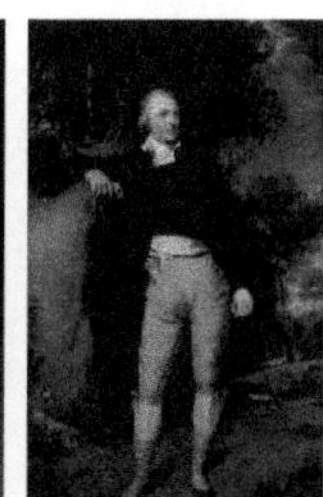
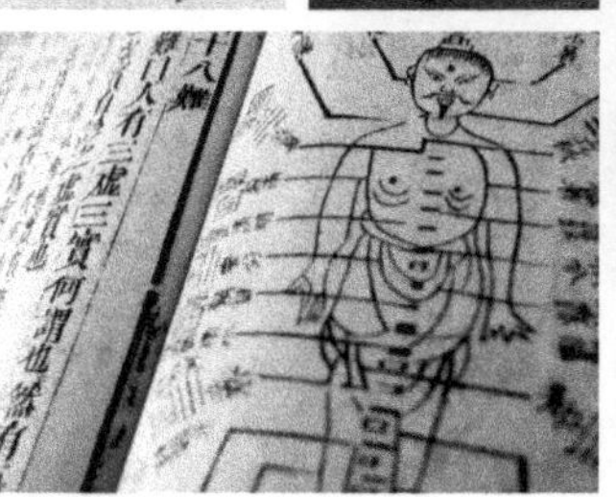
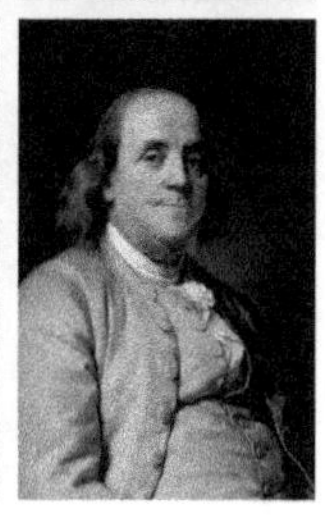

CHAPTER 3
THE KEY PURPOSE AND WHY

The Key Purpose and Why

Catheterisation is a medical procedure with several critical purposes that make it indispensable in healthcare. Understanding these purposes helps us appreciate why catheterisation is not just a technical procedure but a vital aspect of patient care that enhances both physical health and quality of life. In this chapter, we will explore the primary reasons for catheterisation, including urinary drainage and relief from urinary retention, diagnostic and surgical applications, and the enhancement of patient dignity and comfort.

Urinary Drainage and Relief from Urinary Retention

At its core, catheterisation is about ensuring that urine is efficiently and effectively drained from the bladder. Urinary

Enhancing Patient Dignity and Comfort

While the technical aspects of catheterisation are essential, it is equally important to consider the human element.

Catheterisation, when done correctly and with empathy, significantly enhances patient dignity and comfort.

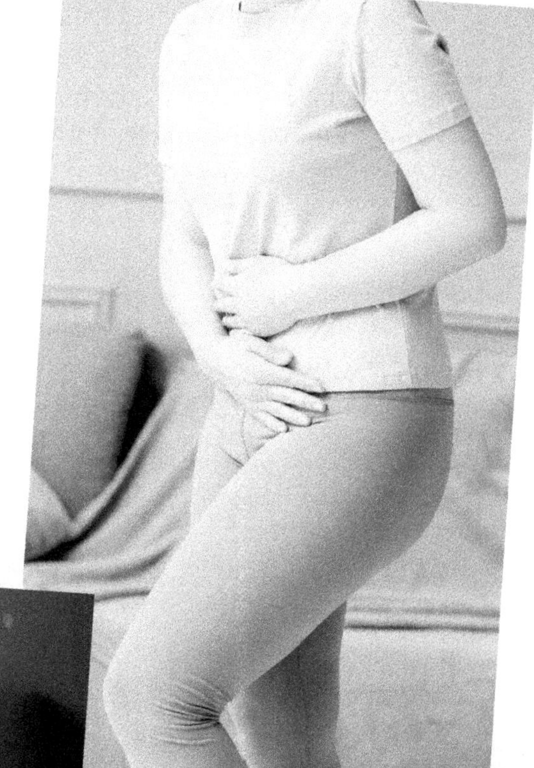

Urinary Retention: Causes and Consequences

Urinary retention can occur for a variety of reasons, including:

- **Obstructions:** Conditions such as benign prostatic hyperplasia (BPH) in men, urethral strictures, or kidney stones can block the flow of urine.
- **Nerve-related Issues:** Neurological disorders like spinal cord injuries, multiple sclerosis, or diabetes can interfere with the nerves that control bladder function.
- **Medications:** Certain medications can impair bladder function as a side effect.
- **Post-Surgical Complications:** Anaesthesia and surgical procedures, particularly those involving the lower abdomen or pelvis, can temporarily disrupt normal bladder function.

If left untreated, urinary retention can lead to bladder damage, urinary tract infections (UTIs), and kidney damage due to backflow of urine into the kidneys. Catheterisation provides immediate relief by allowing urine to bypass the obstruction or dysfunctional bladder, preventing these serious complications.

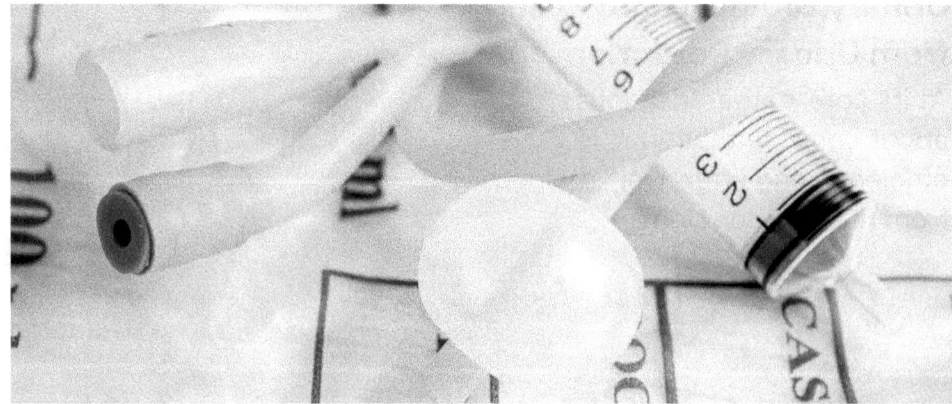

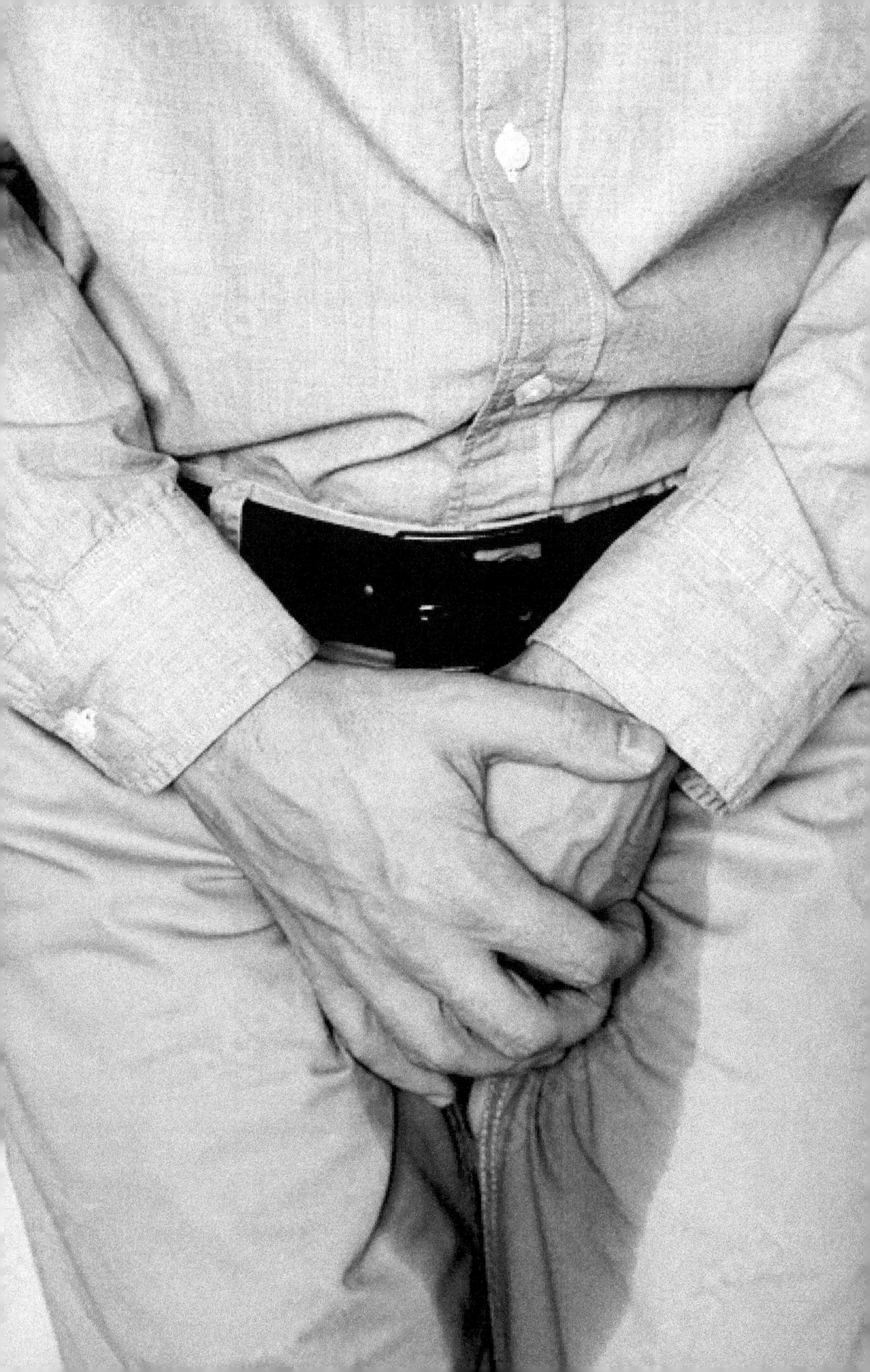

Restoring Dignity

For many patients, issues related to urinary retention or incontinence can be profoundly embarrassing and distressing. Catheterisation helps restore a sense of normalcy and dignity:

- **Managing Incontinence:** For patients who experience urinary incontinence, catheters offer a reliable solution that prevents the embarrassment of accidents and allows them to participate in daily activities without fear.
- **Post-Surgical Recovery:** After surgery, patients are often vulnerable and in discomfort. Catheterisation ensures that urinary needs are met discreetly, allowing patients to focus on recovery without additional stress.

Improving Comfort

Comfort is a critical aspect of patient care, and catheterisation can play a significant role in enhancing it:

- **Relieving Discomfort:** Urinary retention can cause significant pain and discomfort. By providing immediate relief, catheters improve the patient's overall sense of well-being.
- **Minimizing Infections:** Modern catheter designs and techniques emphasize infection prevention. Antimicrobial coatings, sterile insertion procedures, and closed drainage systems reduce the risk of catheter-associated urinary tract infections (CAUTIs), contributing to patient comfort and safety.
- **Customized Care:** Advances in catheter technology mean that patients can receive catheters tailored to their specific needs. From different sizes and materials to options like intermittent or indwelling catheters, customization ensures maximum comfort and effectiveness.

Empowering Patients

Empowering patients is paramount in today's healthcare landscape for several compelling reasons. Firstly, it fosters a sense of autonomy and control over one's own health journey, instilling confidence, and a proactive mindset. When patients feel empowered, they're more likely to engage in shared decision-making with their healthcare providers, leading to better treatment adherence and outcomes. Additionally, empowerment enhances patient satisfaction and overall experience, as individuals feel valued and respected in their care. Moreover, empowered patients are better equipped to navigate complex healthcare systems, advocating for their needs and rights effectively. Ultimately, by empowering patients, we not only improve individual health outcomes but also contribute to a more patient-centred and efficient healthcare system as a whole.

Education and support are key to successful catheterization:

- **Self-Catheterisation**: For patients who can perform intermittent catheterisation themselves, training and resources empower them to manage their condition independently. This autonomy boosts confidence and reduces dependency on caregivers.
- **Patient Education:** Clear instructions, support from healthcare providers, and access to resources such as videos and guides help patients understand and manage their catheter care effectively.

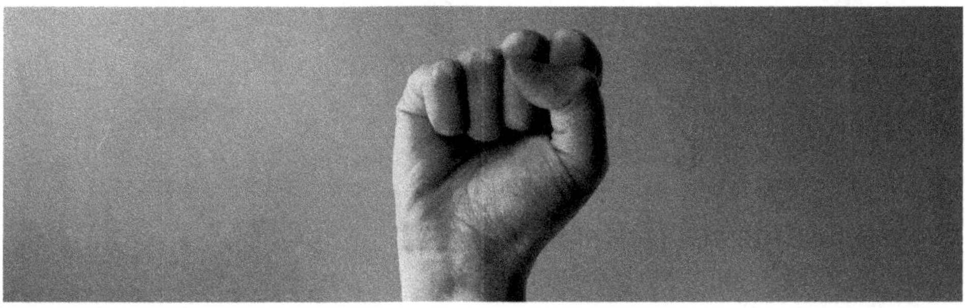

Conclusion

Catheterisation is a multifaceted medical procedure with purposes that go far beyond simple urinary drainage. Its ability to relieve urinary retention, facilitate diagnostic and surgical procedures, and enhance patient dignity and comfort makes it a cornerstone of effective healthcare.

By understanding the key purposes of catheterisation, caregivers and healthcare providers can approach this procedure with the knowledge and empathy needed to provide the best possible care. In the next chapters, we will delve deeper into the methods and types of catheterisations, what to look for in catheter care, maintaining personal hygiene and dignity, and handy tips for keeping accurate records.

Together, we will build a comprehensive understanding of how to manage catheter care with compassion and competence, ensuring that every patient can go with dignity and comfort.

MAINTAINING PERSONAL HYGIENE

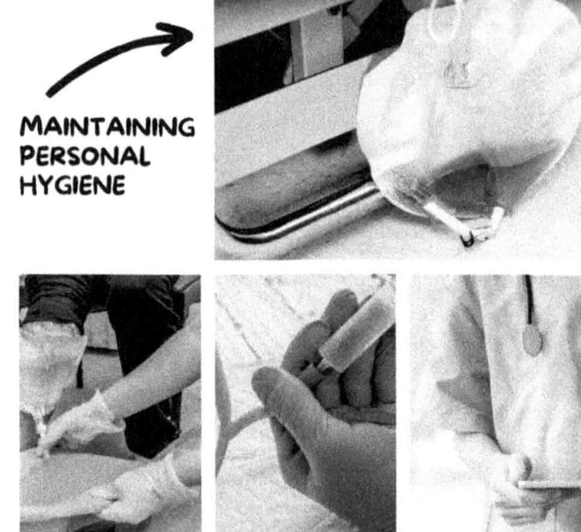

BRINGS DIGNITY AND EMPOWERMENT

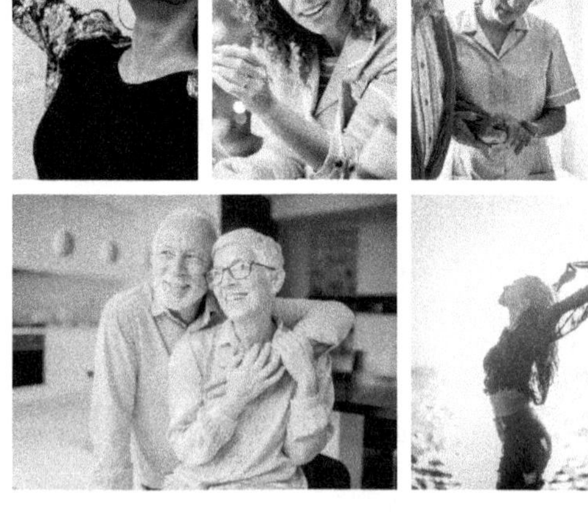

CHAPTER 4
THE METHODS AND TYPES OF CATHETERS

Methods of Catheterisation

Catheterisation involves different techniques depending on the patient's needs, medical conditions, and the intended duration of use. The primary methods include intermittent catheterisation, indwelling catheterisation (Foley), suprapubic catheterisation, and external (condom) catheterisation.

Intermittent Catheterisation

Intermittent catheterisation involves the periodic insertion of a catheter to drain urine from the bladder. This method is often used by individuals who need to empty their bladders at regular intervals but do not require a permanent catheter.

- **Procedure:** The catheter is inserted into the urethra, urine is drained, and then the catheter is removed. This process is typically repeated several times a day.

- **Advantages:** Intermittent catheterisation reduces the risk of infection compared to indwelling catheters because the catheter is not constantly in place. It also allows for greater mobility and comfort.

- **Uses:** It is commonly used by patients with chronic urinary retention, spinal cord injuries, or neurogenic bladder conditions.

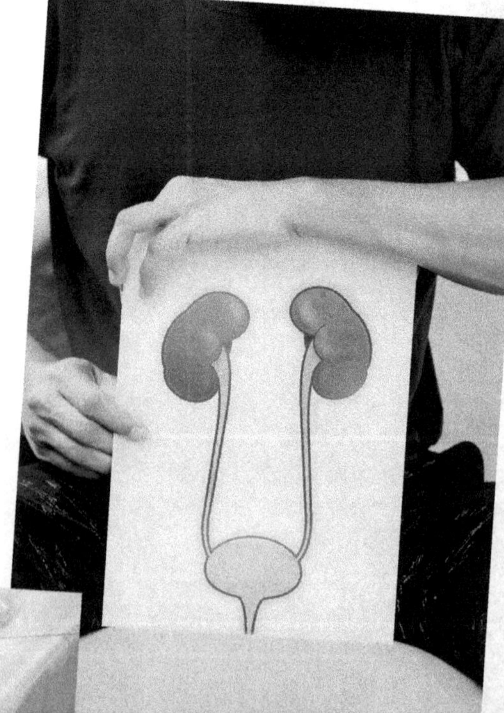

Indwelling Catheterisation (Foley Catheter)

Indwelling catheters, also known as Foley catheters, are designed to remain in the bladder for an extended period. They are often used when continuous drainage is necessary.

- **Procedure:** The catheter is inserted into the urethra and advanced into the bladder. A small balloon at the tip is then inflated to keep the catheter in place.
- **Advantages:** This method provides continuous drainage, which is essential for patients who are bedridden, undergoing surgery, or have significant mobility issues.
- **Uses:** Indwelling catheters are used in patients with urinary retention, severe incontinence, during and after surgery, and in those who are unable to self-catheterise.

Suprapubic Catheterisation

Suprapubic catheterisation involves the insertion of a catheter through a small incision in the lower abdomen directly into the bladder. This method is an alternative to urethral catheterisation.

- **Procedure:** A minor surgical procedure is performed to place the catheter through the abdominal wall into the bladder.
- **Advantages:** Suprapubic catheters reduce the risk of urethral trauma and infection. They are often more comfortable for long-term use and allow for normal sexual activity.
- **Uses:** This method is suitable for patients with urethral blockages, long-term catheterisation needs, or those who have had previous pelvic surgeries.

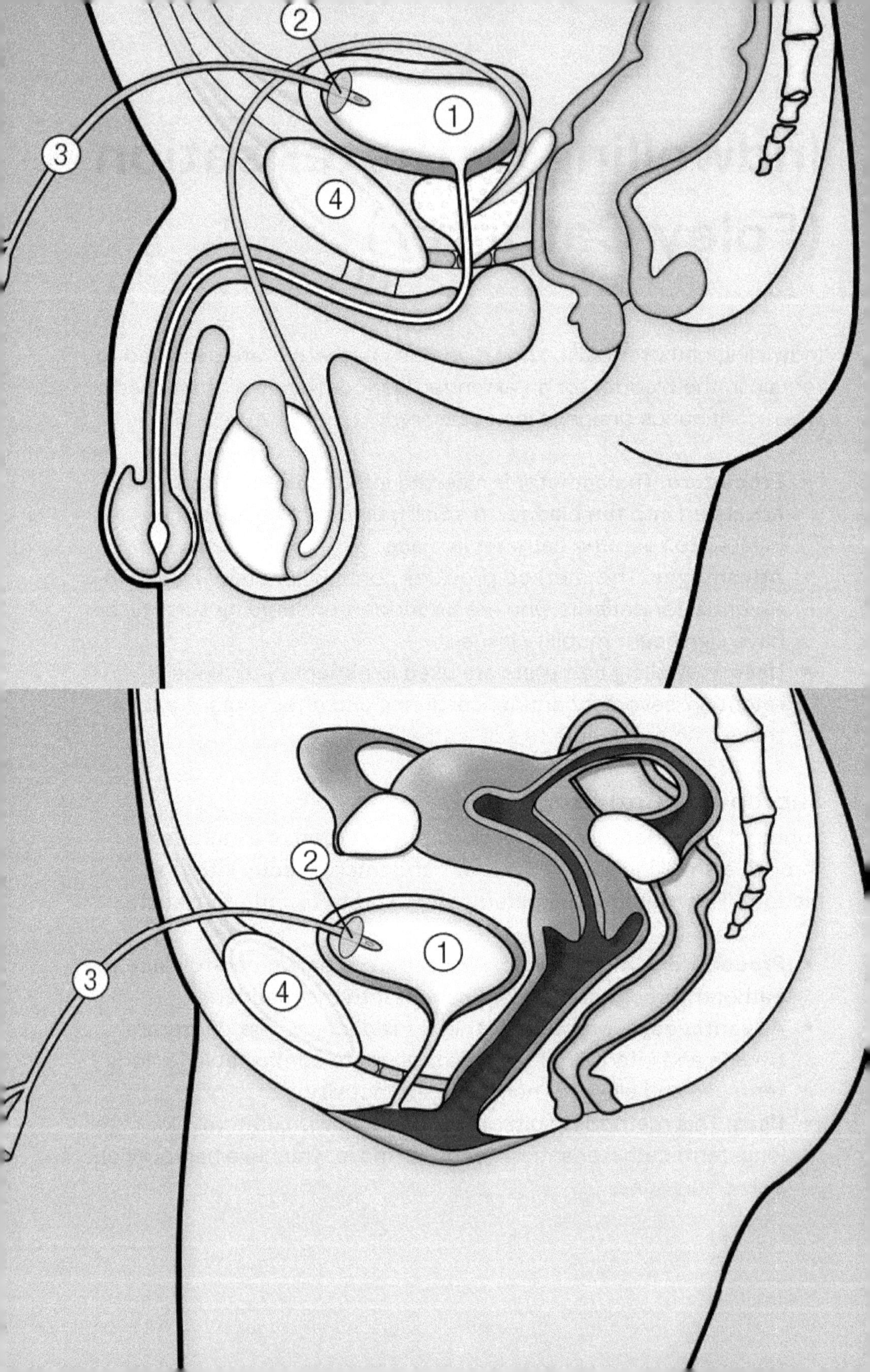

External (Condom) Catherisation

External catheters, commonly known as condom catheters, are non-invasive and fit over the penis to collect urine. They are also known as conveens.

- **Procedure:** The catheter is placed over the penis like a condom and connected to a drainage bag.
- **Advantages**: This method is less invasive, reducing the risk of infection and urethral injury. It is also more comfortable for some patients.
- **Uses:** External catheters are primarily used in male patients with incontinence who do not have urinary retention or significant bladder dysfunction.

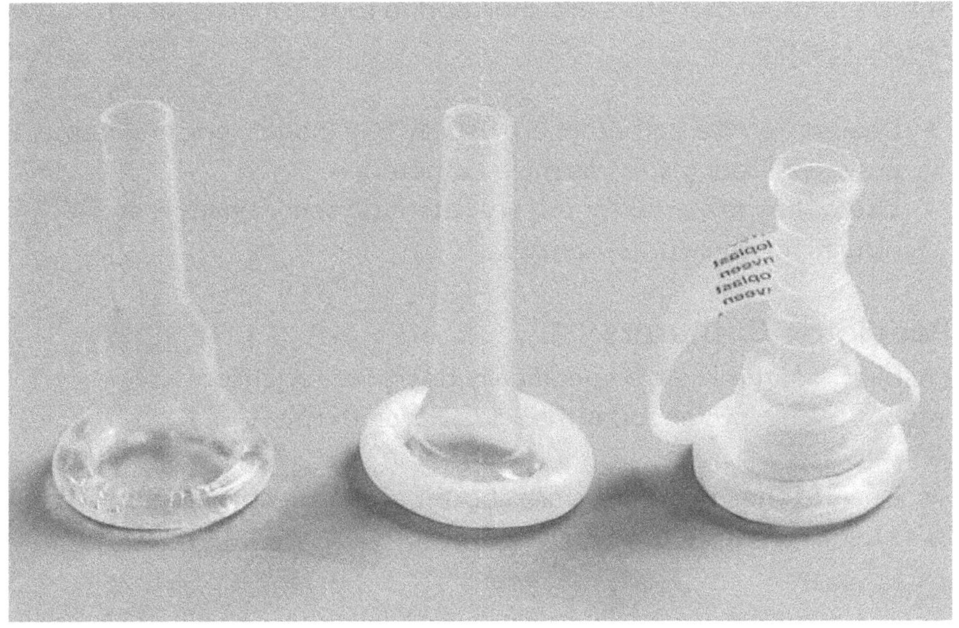

Types of Catheters

Different types of catheters are designed to meet the specific needs of various patient populations, including male, female, paediatric patients, and those requiring specialized catheters like two-way and three-way catheters.

Male Urethral Catheters

Male urethral catheters are typically longer than female catheters to accommodate the male urethra's length.

- **Design:** These catheters are usually 16–18 inches long and come in various sizes measured in French units (Fr).
- **Uses:** They are used for urinary retention, incontinence, and post-surgical drainage.

Female Urethral Catheters

Female urethral catheters are shorter due to the shorter length of the female urethra.

- **Design:** Female catheters are usually 6–8 inches long and come in similar French sizes as male catheters.
- **Uses:** They are used for urinary retention, incontinence, and obtaining sterile urine samples.

Paediatric Catheters

Paediatric catheters are specifically designed for children and infants, taking into account their smaller anatomy.

- **Design:** These catheters are shorter and have smaller diameters, typically ranging from 6 Fr to 12 Fr.

- **Uses:** Paediatric catheters are used in children for urinary retention, congenital abnormalities, and after certain surgeries.

Two-Way and Three-Way Catheters

Two-way and three-way catheters have additional features to facilitate various medical needs.

- **Two-Way Catheters:** These catheters have two channels (lumens): one for draining urine and one for inflating the balloon that holds the catheter in place.
- **Uses**: Commonly used for standard indwelling catheterization where continuous drainage is needed.
- **Three-Way Catheters:** These catheters have a third channel for irrigation, allowing fluids to be flushed into the bladder.
- **Uses:** Often used after bladder or prostate surgery to prevent blood clots from blocking the catheter.

Sizes and Appropriate Use

Catheter sizes are measured in French units (Fr), with the size indicating the external diameter of the catheter. Selecting the appropriate size is crucial for patient comfort and effective drainage.

- **Adult Males:** Typically use catheters ranging from 14 Fr to 18 Fr. The choice depends on the individual's anatomy and the specific clinical situation.
- **Adult Females:** Typically use catheters ranging from 12 Fr to 16 Fr. As with males, the choice depends on comfort and effectiveness.
- **Paediatric Patients:** Catheters for children usually range from 6 Fr to 12 Fr, depending on the child's age and size.

Choosing the correct size is essential to ensure that the catheter is effective and minimizes discomfort and complications. A catheter that is too large can cause pain and urethral trauma, while one that is too small may not drain urine effectively.

Conclusion

Understanding the various methods and types of catheterisations, as well as the appropriate sizes and uses, is vital for caregivers and healthcare providers. Each method and type of catheter serves a specific purpose and is chosen based on the patient's individual needs and medical conditions. By selecting the appropriate catheter and method, we can ensure that patients receive the best possible care, maintain their dignity, and improve their overall quality of life.

In a later chapter, we will discuss the practical aspects of catheter care, including what to look for in terms of signs of complications and how to maintain personal hygiene and dignity for patients undergoing catheterisation.

This knowledge will further equip you to provide compassionate and competent care, ensuring that patients can go with dignity and comfort.

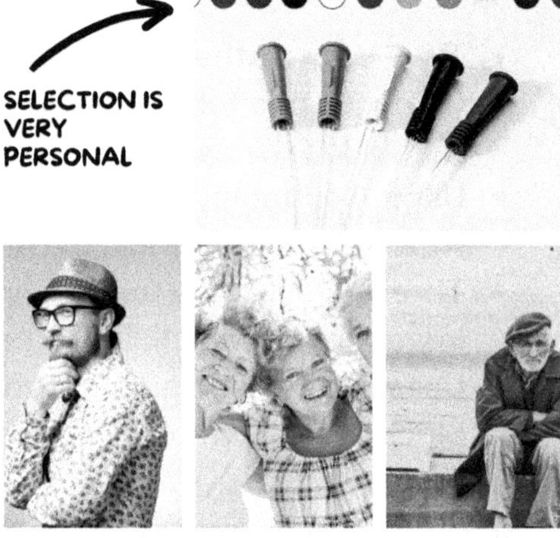

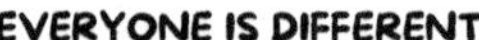

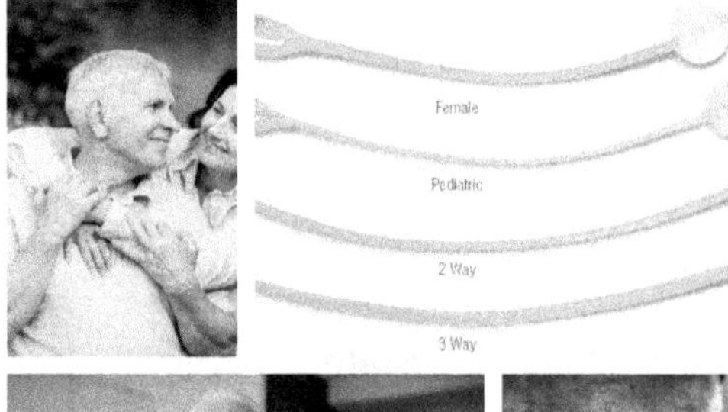

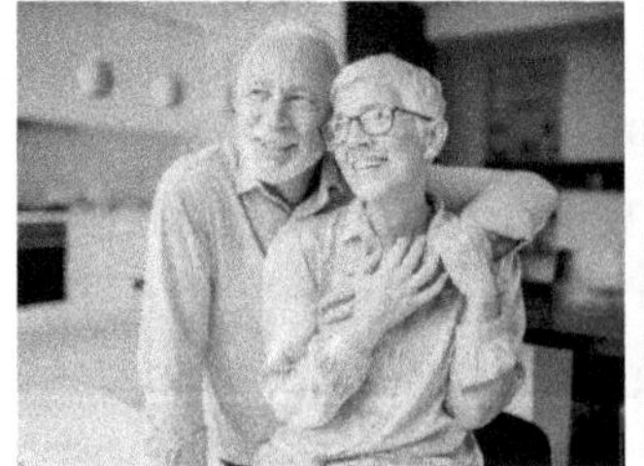

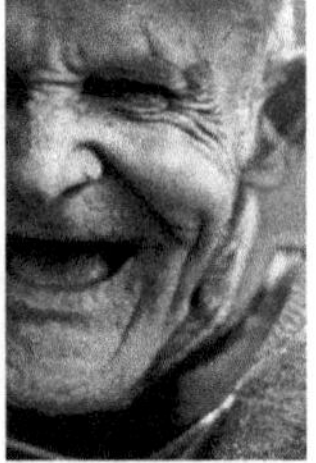

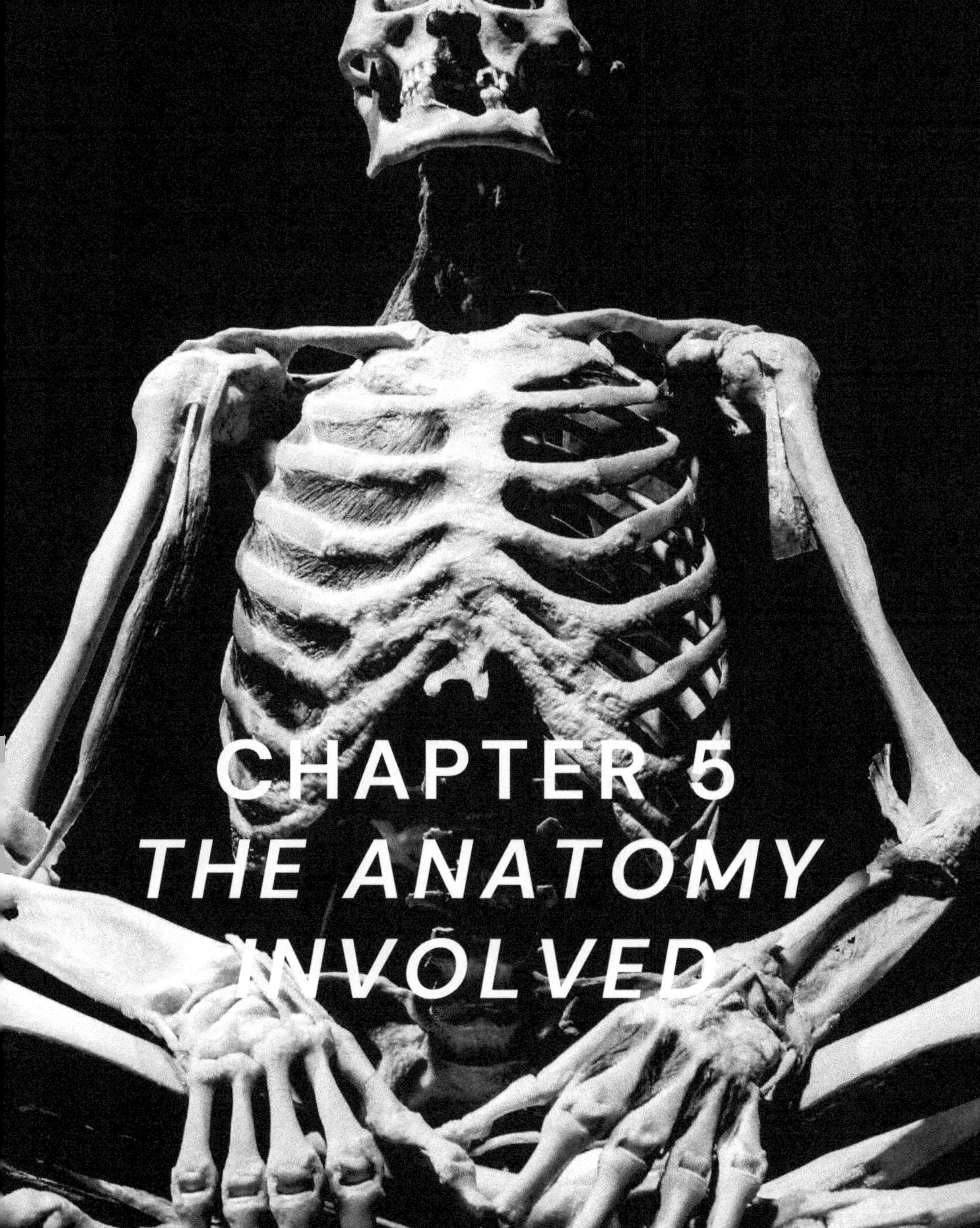
CHAPTER 5
THE ANATOMY
INVOLVED

The Anatomy Involved

In this chapter, we delve into the intricate anatomy of the urinary system, exploring its structure and the differences between male and female anatomy relevant to catheterisation. Understanding the anatomy involved is essential for caregivers and healthcare providers to perform catheteriSation procedures safely and effectively, ensuring optimal patient care and comfort.

Structure of the Urinary System

The urinary system, also known as the renal system, consists of several organs that work together to produce, store, and eliminate urine. Its primary components include the kidneys, ureters, bladder, and urethra.

1. Kidneys

The kidneys are bean-shaped organs located in the retroperitoneal space, one on each side of the spine. They play a crucial role in filtering waste

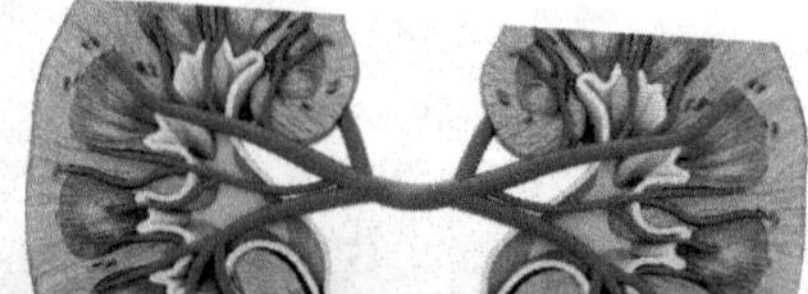

products and excess fluids from the blood to produce urine.

- **Renal Cortex and Medulla:** The outer layer of the kidney is called the renal cortex, while the inner region is known as the renal medulla. These regions contain nephrons, the functional units of the kidneys responsible for urine production.

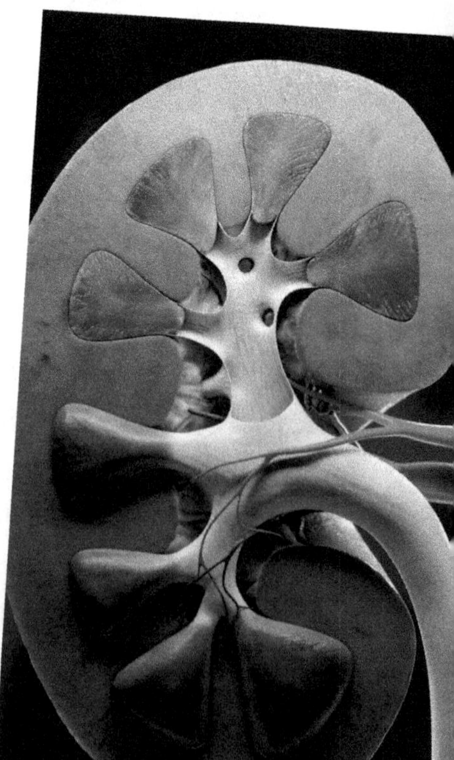

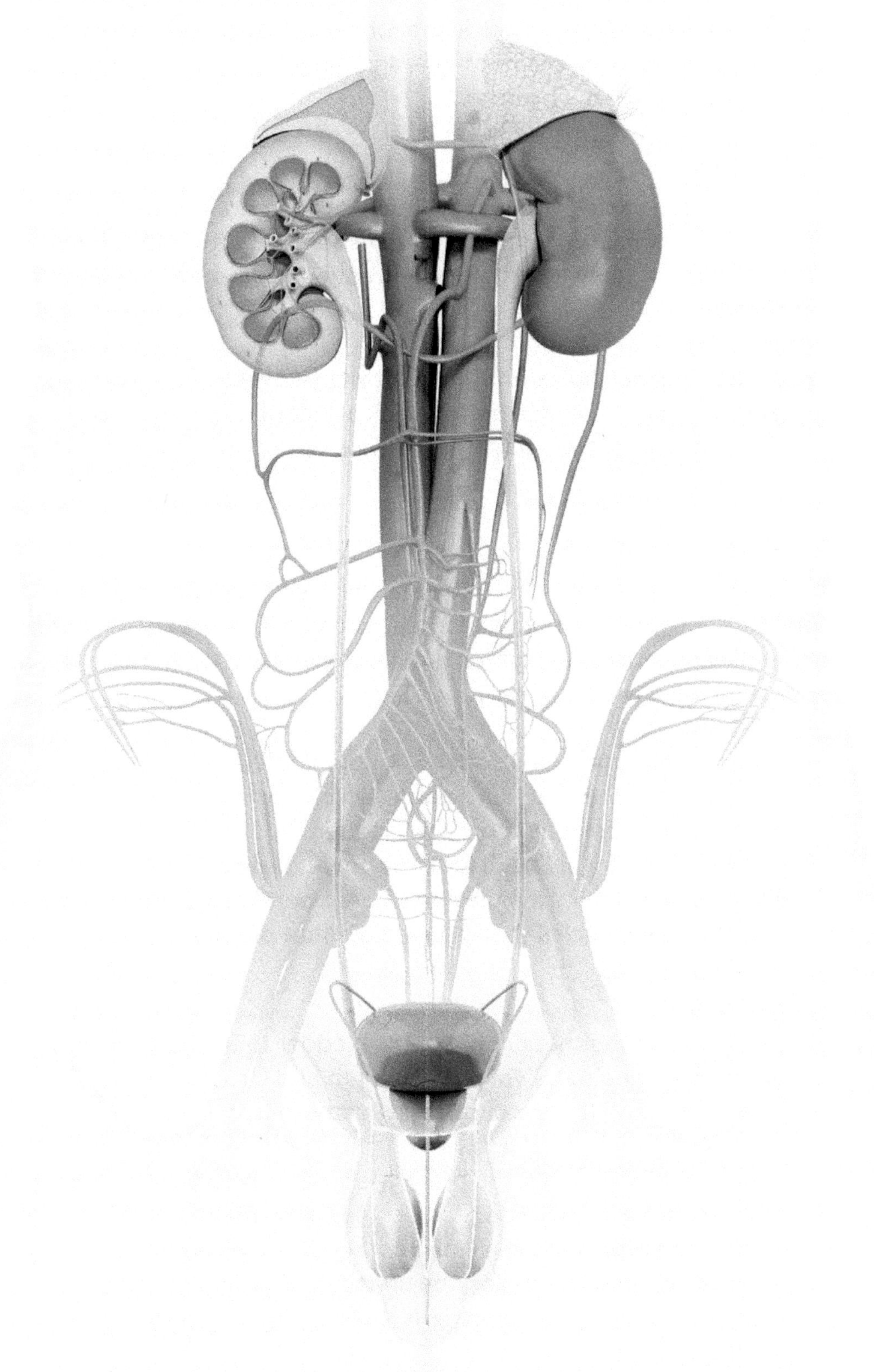

- **Renal Pelvis:** The renal pelvis is a funnel-shaped structure that collects urine from the nephrons and funnels it into the ureters for transport to the bladder.

2. Ureters

The ureters are muscular tubes that connect the kidneys to the bladder. Their primary function is to transport urine from the kidneys to the bladder through peristaltic contractions of the smooth muscle in their walls.

- **Ureterovesical Junction:** The point where the ureter enters the bladder is known as the ureterovesical junction. It is equipped with one-way valves that prevent urine from flowing back into the kidneys.

3. Bladder

The bladder is a hollow, muscular organ located in the pelvis that serves as a reservoir for urine storage. Its capacity can vary depending on individual factors, but it can typically hold approximately 400–600 millilitres of urine.

- **Detrusor Muscle:** The bladder wall contains a layer of smooth muscle called the detrusor muscle, which contracts during urination to expel urine from the bladder.
- **Urethral Openings:** The bladder has two openings for the ureters and one opening for the urethra. These openings are controlled by sphincter muscles that regulate the flow of urine.

4. Urethra

The urethra is a tube that connects the bladder to the exterior of the body, allowing urine to be voided. Its length and structure differ between males and females, impacting catheterisation procedures.

- **Male Urethra:** In males, the urethra is longer and passes through the prostate gland and penis. It serves a dual function for both urinary and reproductive systems.
- **Female Urethra:** In females, the urethra is shorter and located anterior to the vaginal opening. It is solely dedicated to urinary function.

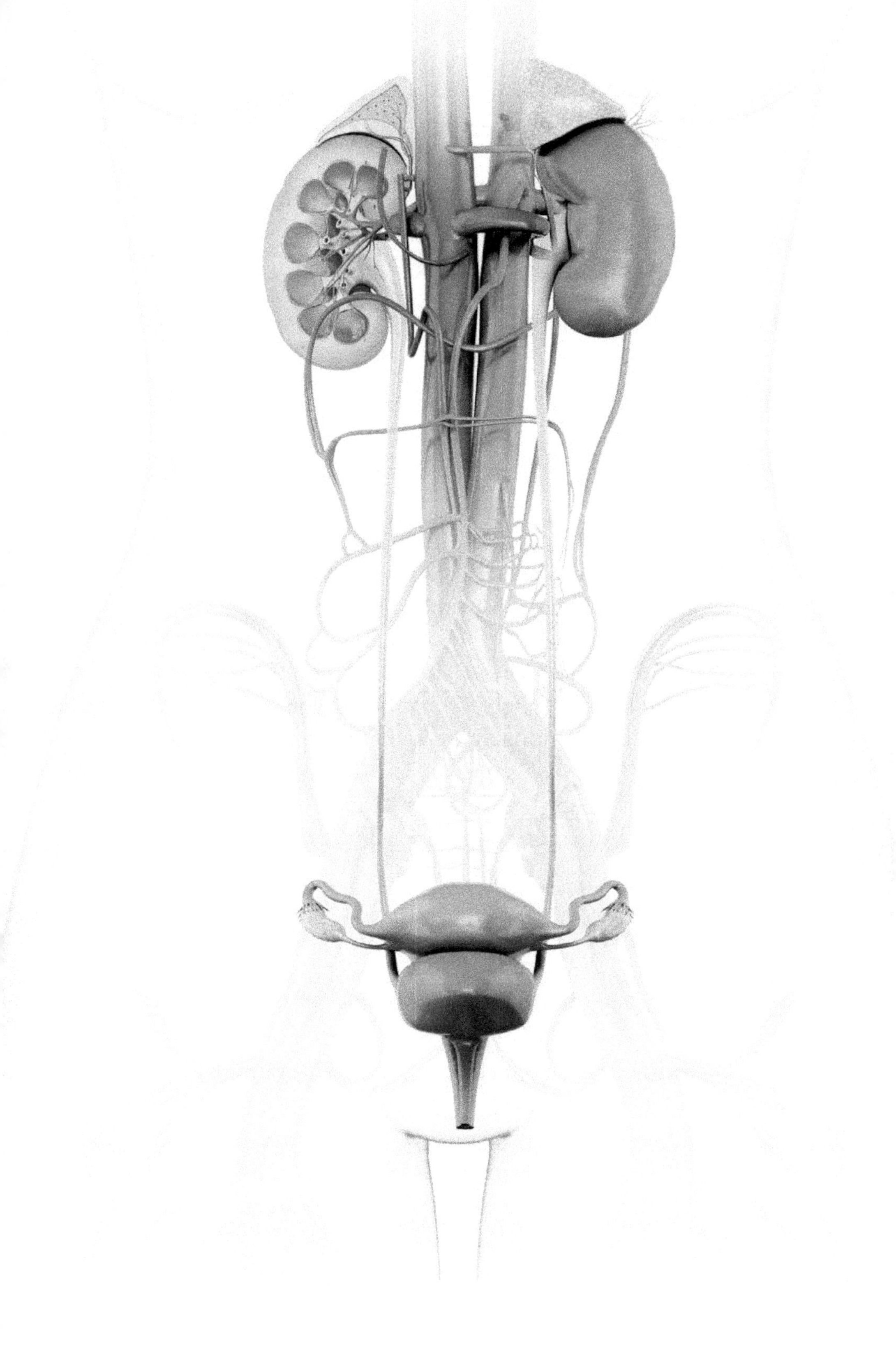

Differences Between Male and Female Anatomy Relevant to Catheterisation

The anatomical differences between male and female urinary systems influence the approach to catheterisation procedures and the selection of catheter types.

1. Male Anatomy

In males, the longer urethra and its passage through the prostate gland present unique considerations for catheterisation:

- **Prostate Gland:** The prostate gland surrounds the urethra just below the bladder. Its proximity to the urethra means that catheter insertion in males requires care to navigate around the gland without causing trauma.
- **Penile Urethra:** The urethra in males passes through the penis, which can affect catheterisation techniques and the choice of catheter size and length.

2. Female Anatomy

Female anatomy differs from males in terms of urethral length and location:

- **Shorter Urethra:** The female urethra is shorter than the male urethra, reducing the distance for catheter insertion. However, its location anterior to the vaginal opening allows for more straightforward access.
- **Absence of Prostate Gland:** Unlike males, females do not have a prostate gland, simplifying catheterisation procedures and reducing the risk of complications related to prostatic obstruction.

Relevance to Catheterisation

Understanding the anatomical nuances of male and female urinary systems is critical for performing catheterisation procedures safely and effectively:

- **Catheter Selection:** Catheters for males may need to be longer to navigate the urethra and pass the prostate gland, while catheters for females can be shorter due to the shorter urethral length.
- **Insertion Technique:** Care must be taken during catheter insertion to minimize trauma to surrounding structures, such as the prostate gland in males or the vaginal wall in females.
- **Complications:** Awareness of anatomical differences helps healthcare providers anticipate and address potential complications, such as urethral trauma or urinary retention, during and after catheterisation.

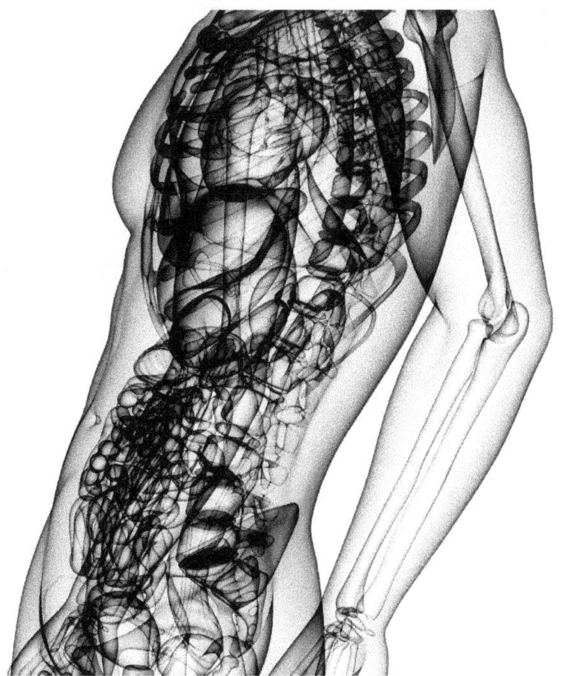

Conclusion

The anatomy of the urinary system, with its intricate structures and physiological functions, plays a crucial role in catheterisation procedures. Understanding the differences between male and female anatomy is essential for selecting appropriate catheters, performing procedures safely, and minimizing the risk of complications.
As caregivers and healthcare providers, a thorough knowledge of urinary system anatomy enables us to provide optimal care and support for patients undergoing catheterisation.

In the next chapter, we will explore practical aspects of catheter care, including maintaining personal hygiene and dignity for patients, and provide handy tips for caregivers to ensure effective catheter management.

With this understanding, we can continue to uphold the principles of compassionate and competent care, ensuring that every patient's needs are met with dignity and respect.

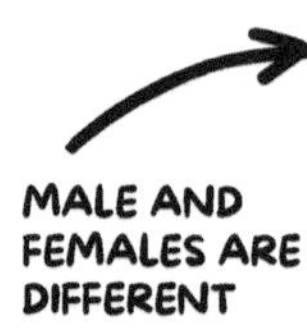

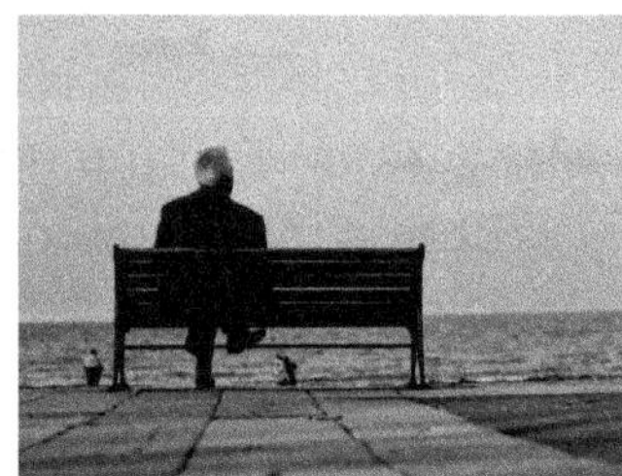
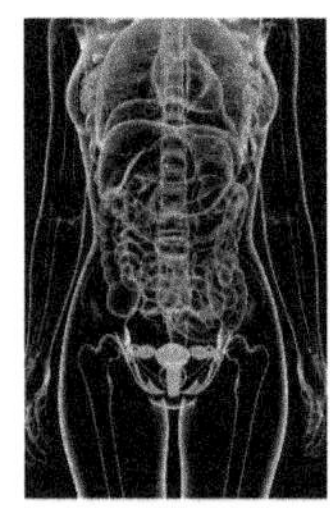
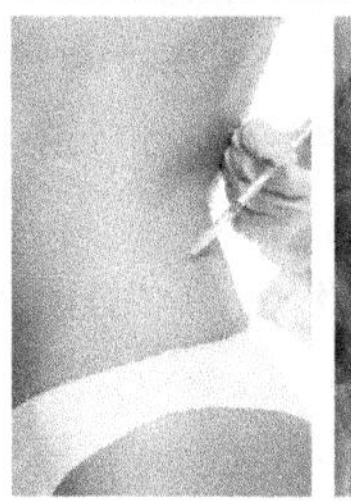
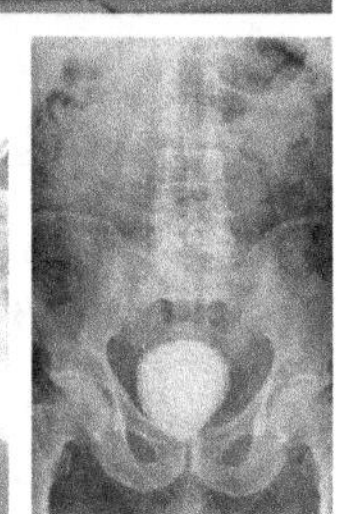

THE URINARY SYSTEM IS IMPORTANT

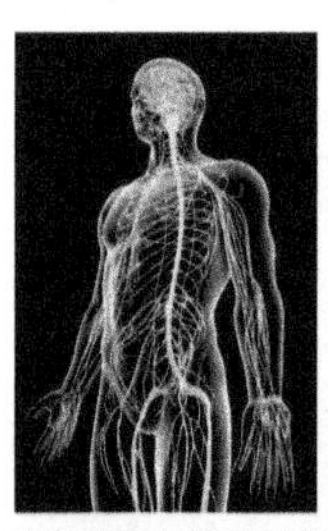
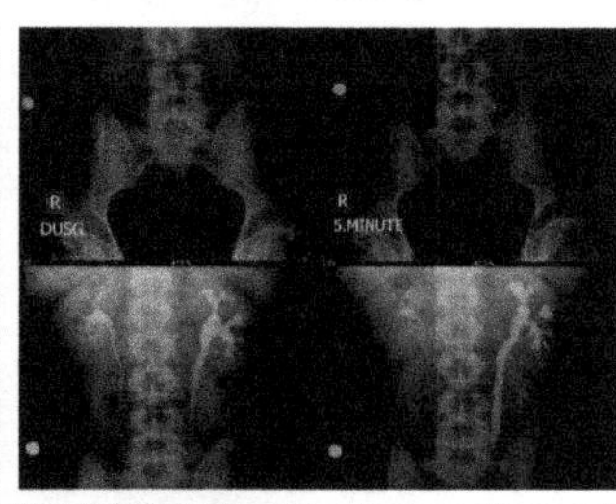
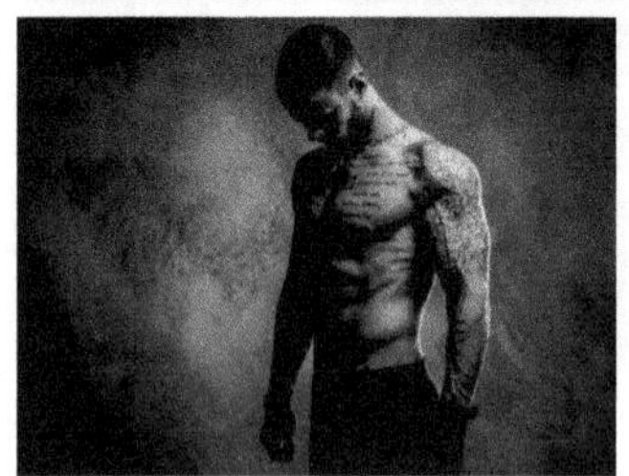
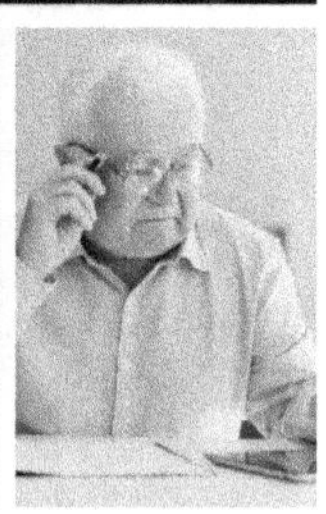

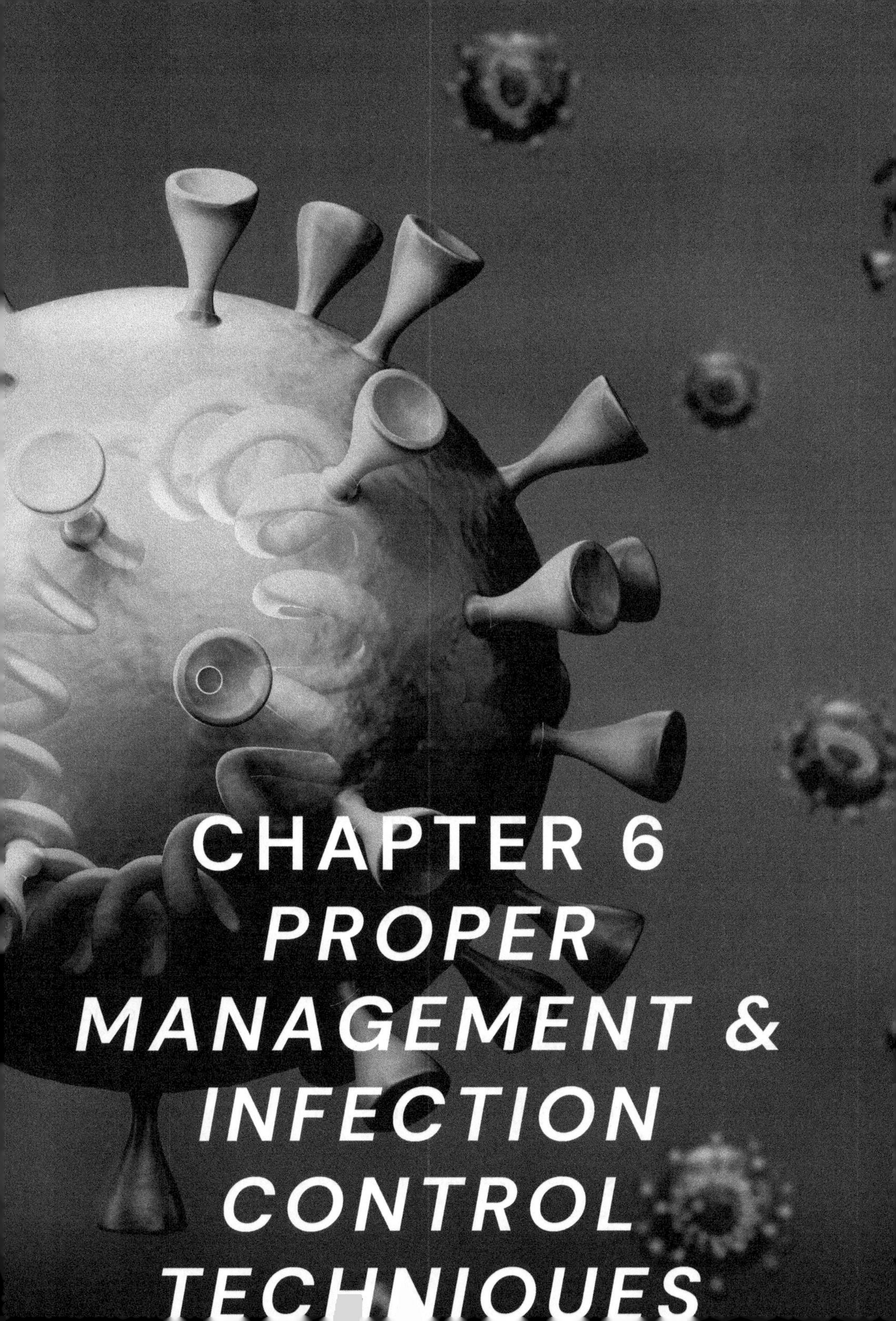
CHAPTER 6
PROPER MANAGEMENT & INFECTION CONTROL TECHNIQUES

Proper Management and Infection Control Techniques

Effective management of catheter bags involves adhering to strict infection control practices and timely maintenance. Here's what caregivers need to know:

1. Changing a Leg Bag: To change a leg bag, follow these steps:

- Wash hands thoroughly with soap and water or use an alcohol-based hand sanitizer.
- Disconnect the old leg bag from the catheter tubing, ensuring a firm grip on both the tubing and the bag to prevent spillage.
- Dispose of the old bag appropriately, following local guidelines for medical waste disposal.
- Clean the catheter tubing connection site with an alcohol wipe or antiseptic solution.
- Connect the new leg bag to the catheter tubing, ensuring a secure fit.
- Secure the new leg bag to the patient's leg using the provided straps or bands, ensuring comfort and proper positioning.

2. When to Empty a Bag: It's crucial to empty catheter bags regularly to prevent overfilling and minimize the risk of urinary tract infections. Caregivers should empty the bag:

- When it's approximately half full or as instructed by healthcare professionals.
- Before bedtime or long periods of rest to ensure uninterrupted drainage and patient comfort.

- Using proper hand hygiene techniques before and after handling the bag and ensuring the drainage spout does not come into contact with any surfaces during emptying.

3. Infection Control Techniques: Infection prevention is paramount in catheter care. Caregivers should:

- Follow strict hand hygiene protocols, washing hands before and after handling catheter bags or performing any catheter-related tasks.
- Clean and disinfect reusable catheter bags regularly using manufacturer-recommended cleaning solutions and techniques.
- Monitor the catheter insertion site for signs of infection, such as redness, swelling, or discharge, and report any abnormalities to healthcare providers promptly.

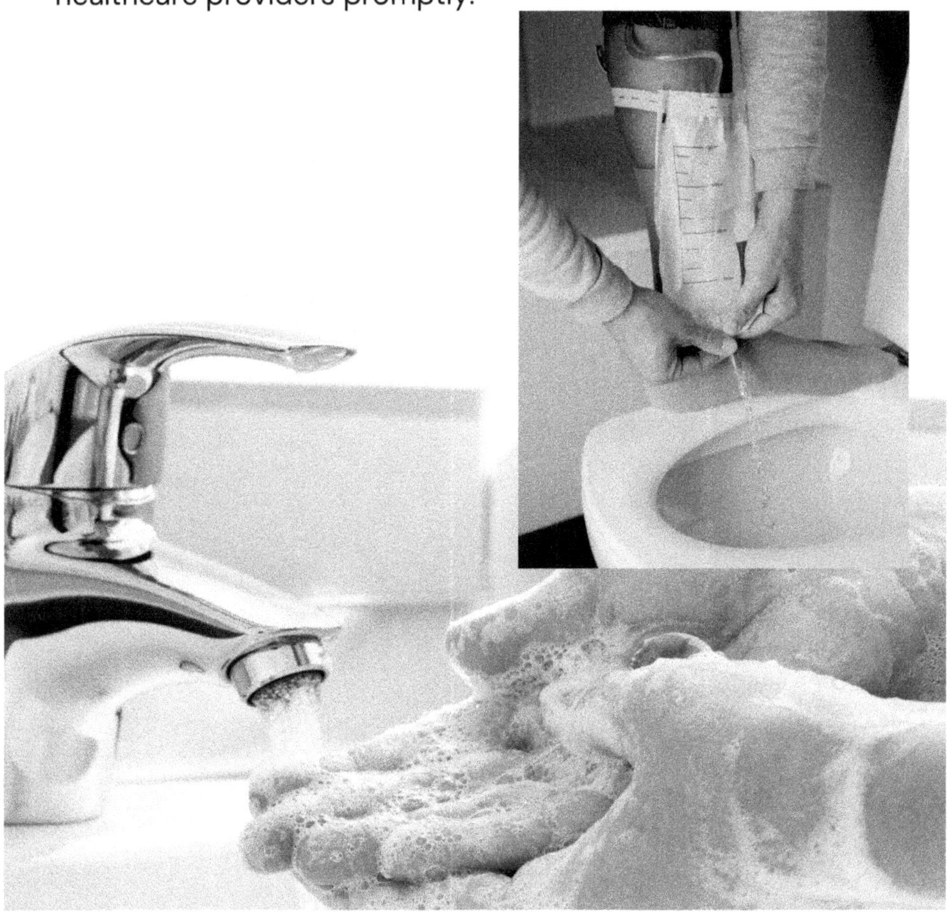

Conclusion

In conclusion, proper management of catheter bags is essential for maintaining patient comfort, hygiene, and overall well-being.

By understanding the different types of catheter bags available and adhering to infection control techniques, caregivers can ensure optimal patient outcomes and minimize the risk of complications.

Effective management of catheter bags not only promotes patient dignity and quality of life but also plays a crucial role in preventing urinary tract infections and other catheter-related complications.

TIP: ALWAYS ensure that the tap is closed when attaching a leg bag or after emptying.

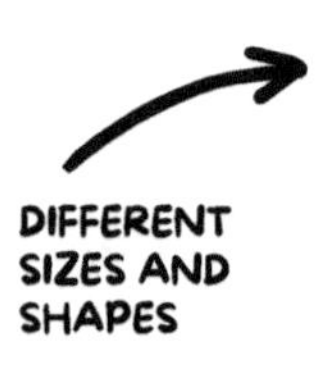

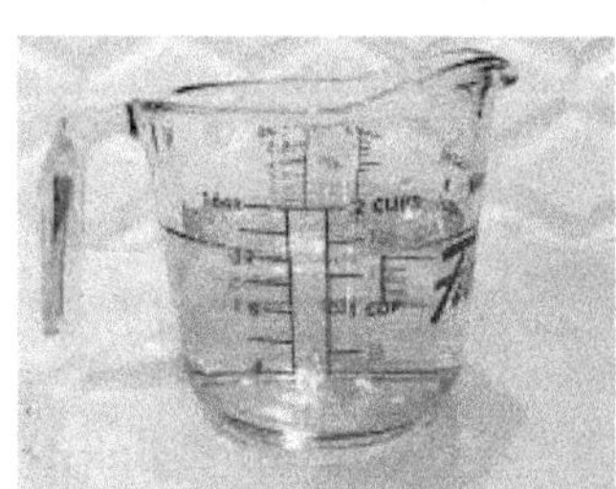

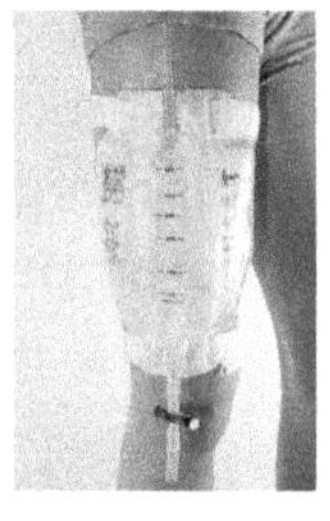

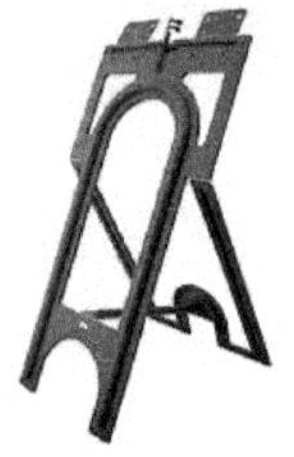

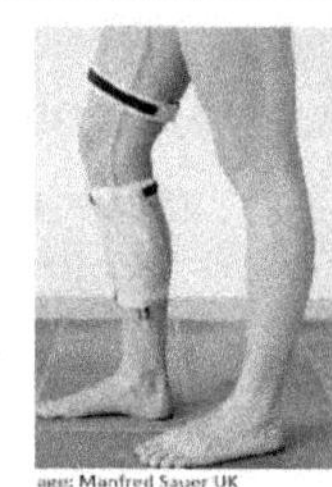

ALWAYS MAKE THE TAP IS CLOSED

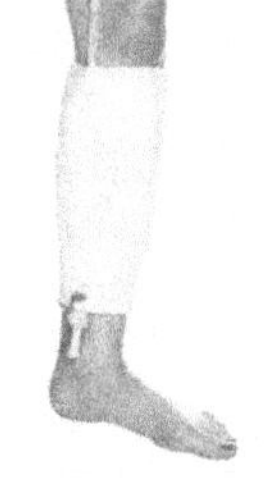

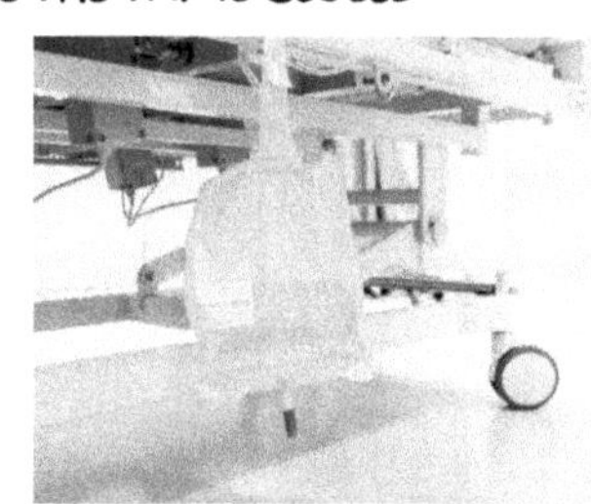

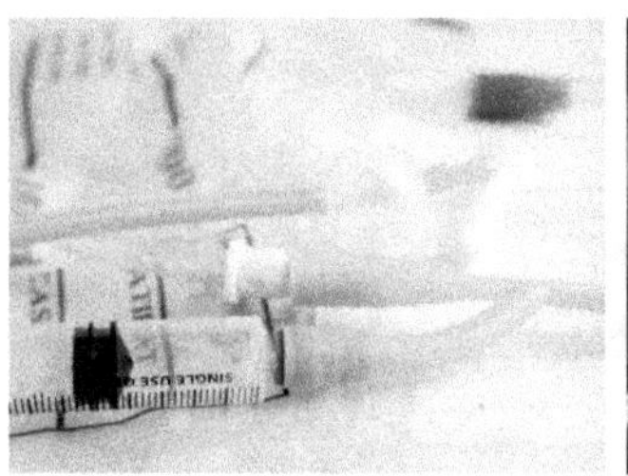

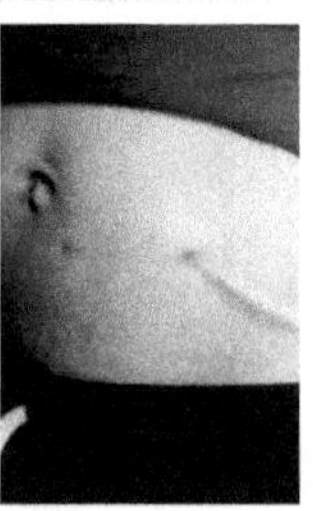

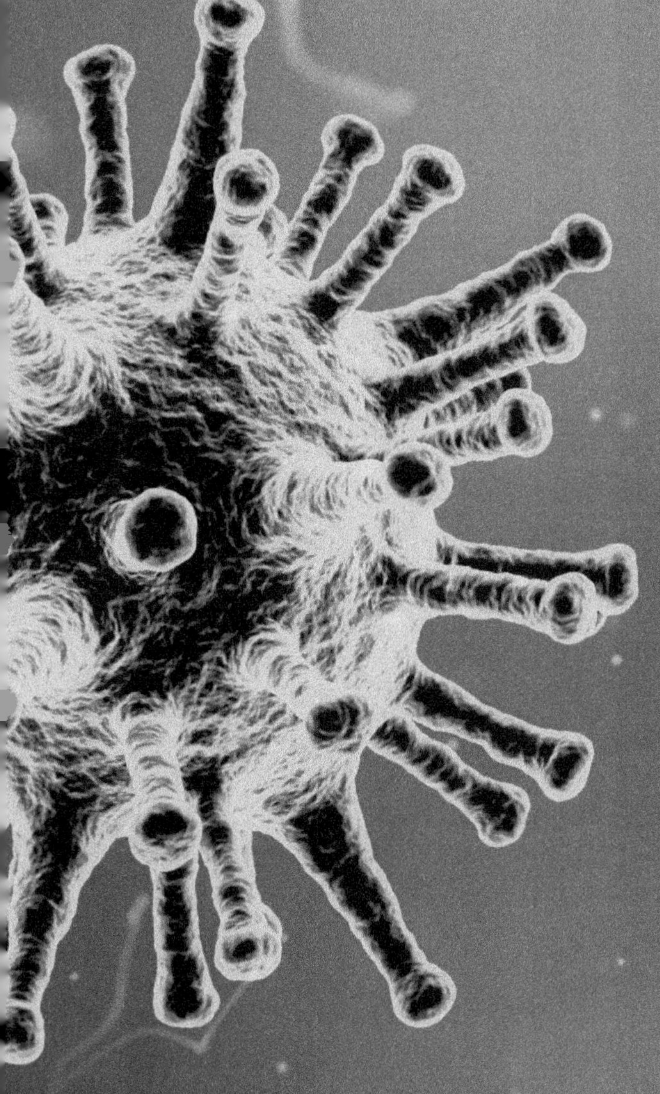

CHAPTER 7
WHAT TO LOOK FOR

Crucial Aspects of Catheter Care

In this chapter, we will discuss crucial aspects of catheter care, focusing on what caregivers and healthcare providers should look for to ensure the safety, comfort, and well-being of patients. This includes recognizing signs of infection or complications, ensuring proper catheter placement and maintenance, and monitoring urine output and quality. Additionally, we'll cover the importance of regular hygiene practices, effective communication with patients about their symptoms and discomfort, and the timely replacement of catheters to prevent long-term issues.

By being vigilant and proactive, we can prevent potential problems and provide the best possible care for patients undergoing catheterisation.

The catheter system should remain closed to avoid infection because a closed system minimizes the risk of bacterial entry. This significantly reduces the likelihood of urinary tract infections, ensuring better patient safety and health outcomes. Consistent vigilance in maintaining a closed system is crucial for preventing complications and promoting patient well-being.

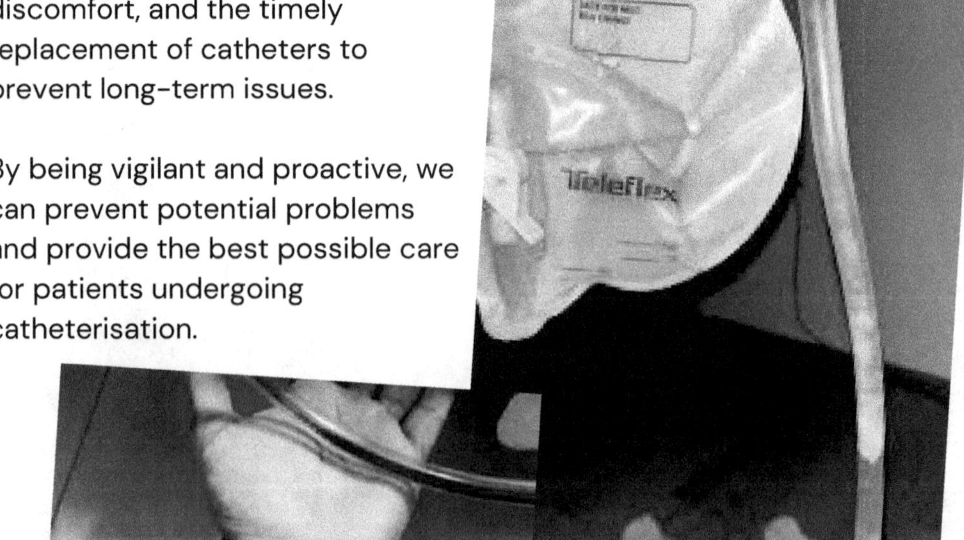

Signs of Infection or Complications

One of the primary concerns in catheter care is the risk of infection or other complications. Caregivers should be vigilant in observing for any signs or symptoms that may indicate a problem. These include:

1. Urinary Tract Infections (UTIs): UTIs are among the most common complications associated with catheterization. Signs of a UTI may include:

- Increased frequency or urgency of urination.
- Pain or burning sensation during urination.
- Cloudy or foul-smelling urine.
- Fever or chills.

2. Catheter-Associated Urinary Tract Infections (CAUTIs): CAUTIs occur when bacteria enter the urinary tract via the catheter. Signs of a CAUTI may include:

- Fever.
- Lower abdominal pain or discomfort.
- Blood in the urine.
- Changes in mental status, particularly in older adults.

3. Blockages or Obstructions: Catheters can become blocked, preventing urine from draining properly. Signs of a blockage may include:

- Decreased or absent urine output.
- Pain or discomfort in the lower abdomen.
- Swelling or leakage around the catheter site.

4. Skin Irritation or Pressure Injuries: Improper catheter placement or inadequate hygiene can lead to skin irritation or pressure injuries around the catheter site. Signs may include:

- Redness, swelling, or tenderness around the catheter insertion site.
- Skin breakdown or ulceration.
- Drainage or leakage of fluid from the insertion site.

Proper Placement and Maintainance

Ensuring proper catheter placement and maintenance is essential for preventing complications and promoting patient comfort. Caregivers should pay close attention to the following aspects:

1. Catheter Insertion:
- Ensure sterile technique during catheter insertion to minimize the risk of infection.
- Confirm proper placement of the catheter tip in the bladder to prevent trauma to the urethra or bladder wall.
- Secure the catheter in place to prevent accidental displacement.

2. Catheter Care:
- Maintain a clean and dry catheter site to reduce the risk of infection and skin irritation.
- Regularly assess the catheter and drainage system for signs of leakage, blockage, or disconnection.
- Empty drainage bags regularly and ensure proper positioning to facilitate drainage.

3. Hygiene Practices:
- Practice proper hand hygiene before and after handling the catheter or drainage system to prevent contamination.
- Clean the periurethral area and catheter insertion site regularly with mild soap and water to maintain hygiene.

Placement Of The Catheter Bag

Ensuring the catheter bag is properly placed is crucial for patient comfort and preventing complications. Here's how to do it correctly:

Securing the Bag:

- For leg bags, use the provided straps or elastic bands to secure the bag to the patient's leg. The bag should be placed lower than the bladder to allow gravity to aid in drainage.
- Ensure the straps are snug but not too tight to prevent circulation issues. Adjust for comfort, avoiding any sharp edges or pressure points.

Locking Mechanism:

- Ensure all locks and connections between the catheter and the bag are securely fastened to prevent leaks and disconnections.
- Double-check that the anti-reflux valve is functioning correctly to avoid urine backflow, which can lead to infections.

Comfort and Safety:

- Periodically check the positioning of the bag and straps to ensure there is no undue pressure or discomfort.
- For men, particular care should be taken to avoid any pulling on the catheter, as this can cause significant pain and injury.

Do Not Leave Tap or Bag Exposed

- Think of dignity. Do not leave tap or bag exposed out of bottom of trousers. Would you want people to see this?

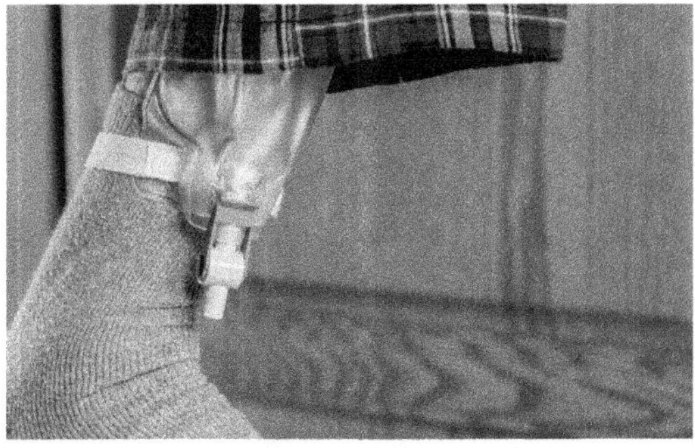

Foley Catheter Female

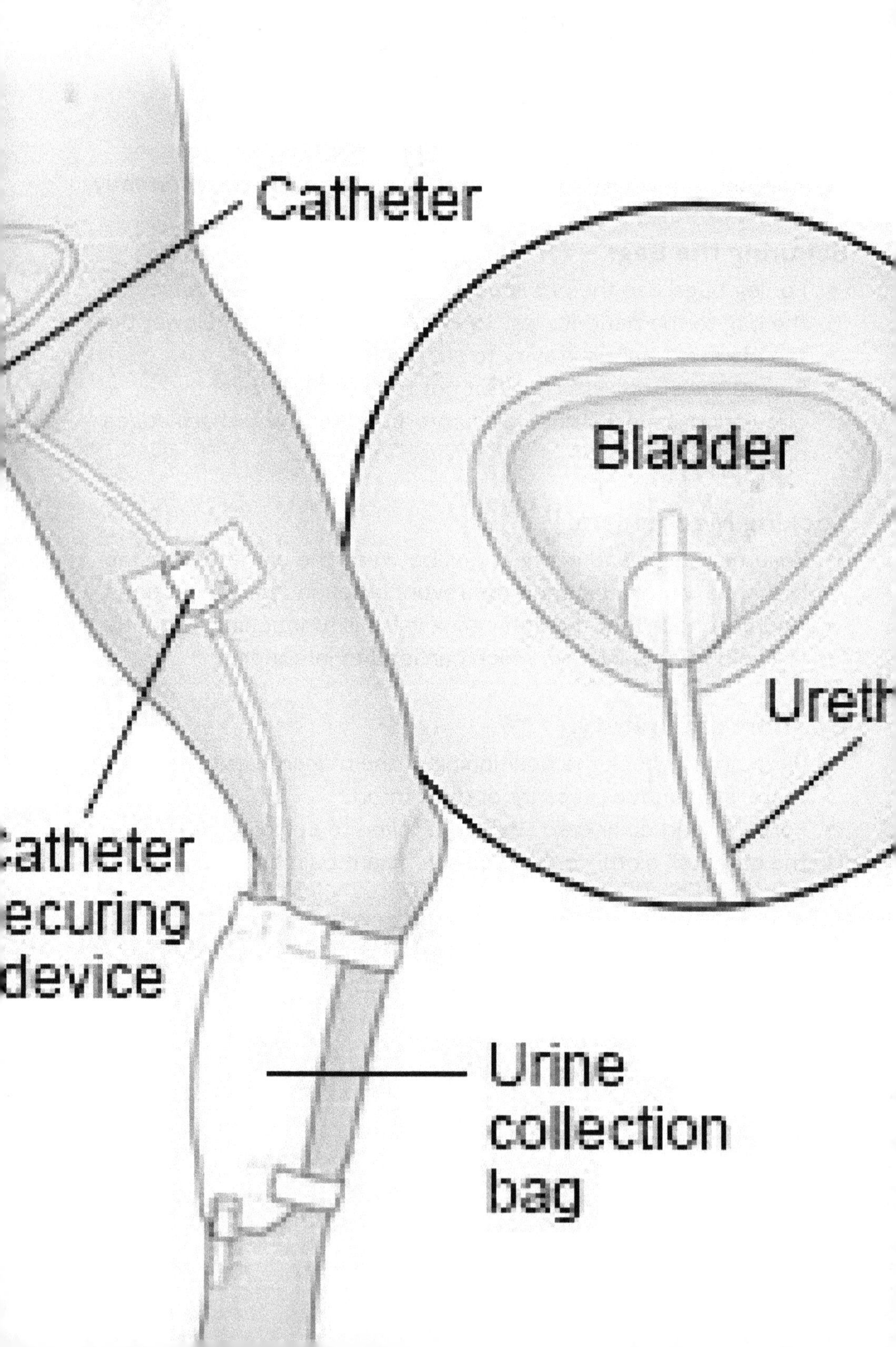

Foley Catheter Male

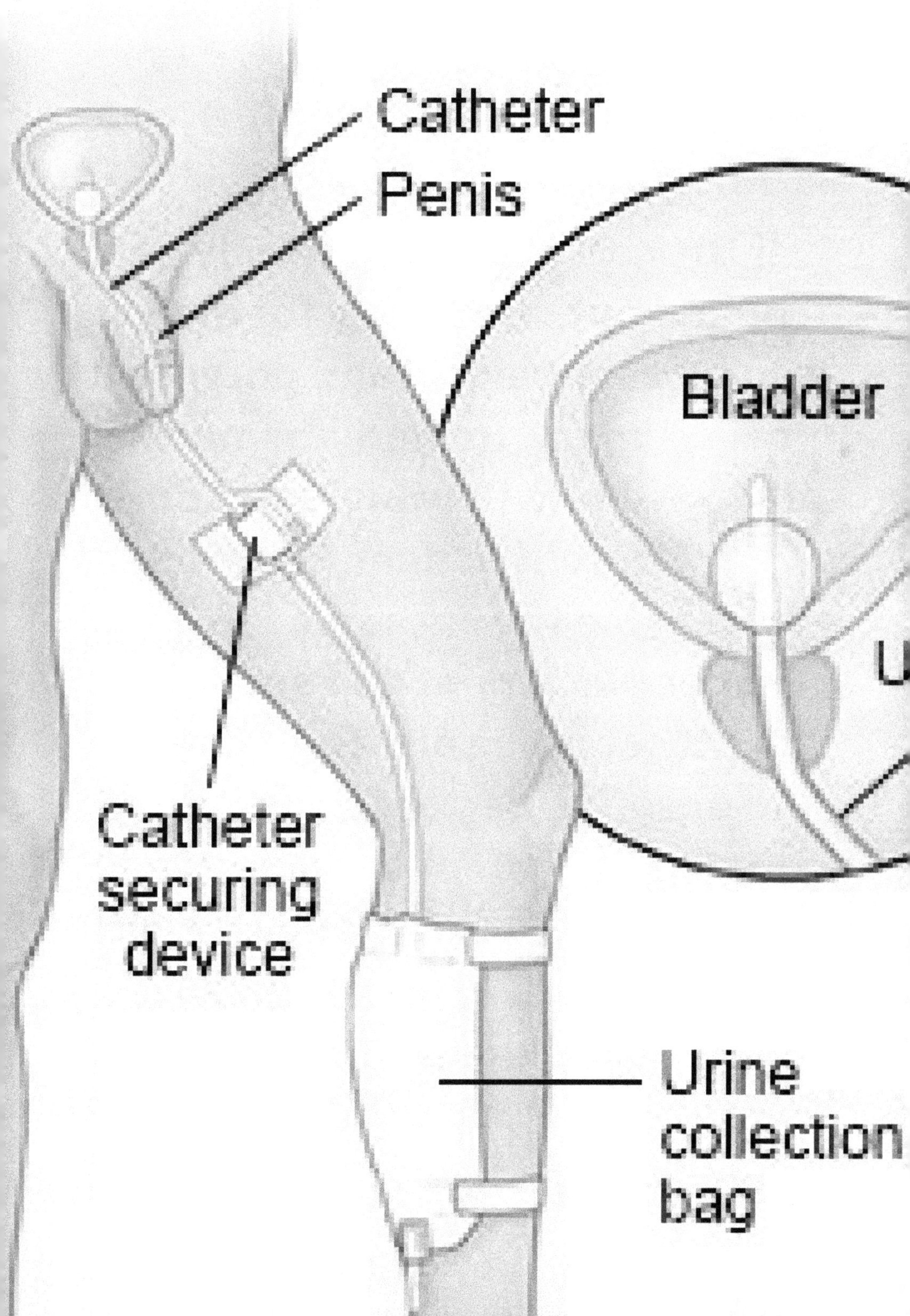

Important Note:

If the catheter accidentally gets pulled out, especially for men, it can be very painful and potentially cause injury. Immediate medical advice should be sought to address any potential damage and to replace the catheter safely. Proper placement and securing of the catheter bag are essential steps in ensuring patient comfort and preventing complications. Always handle the catheter and bag with care to maintain the integrity of the system and the well-being of the patient.

Monitoring Urine Output and Quality

Monitoring urine output and quality is essential for assessing renal function, fluid balance, and the effectiveness of catheterisation. Caregivers should:

1. Measure Urine Output:

- Record the volume and characteristics of urine output regularly to monitor kidney function and fluid status.
- Report any significant changes in urine output, such as sudden increases or decreases, to healthcare providers.

2. Assess Urine Characteristics:

- Observe the colour, clarity, and odour of urine for any abnormalities that may indicate infection or other issues.
- Note any changes in urine colour or odour, such as cloudy or foul-smelling urine, and report them promptly.

3. Monitor for Complications:

- Keep a close watch for signs of complications related to catheterization, such as urinary retention, leakage, or discomfort.
- Report any unusual symptoms or concerns to healthcare providers for further evaluation and management.

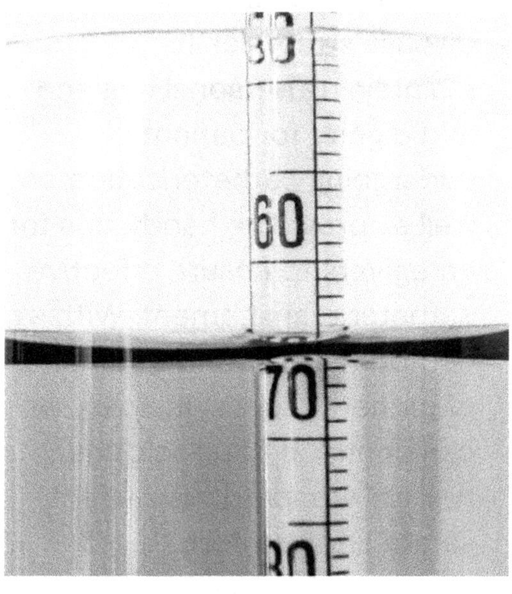

Conclusion

In conclusion, caregivers and healthcare providers play a vital role in ensuring the safety and well-being of patients undergoing catheterisation. By being vigilant and proactive in monitoring for signs of infection or complications, ensuring proper catheter placement and maintenance, and monitoring urine output and quality, we can minimize the risk of complications and provide the best possible care for patients.

In the next chapter, we will discuss strategies for maintaining personal hygiene and dignity for patients undergoing catheterisation, as well as providing handy tips for caregivers to ensure effective catheter management. With a comprehensive understanding of catheter care principles, we can continue to uphold the highest standards of patient safety and comfort.

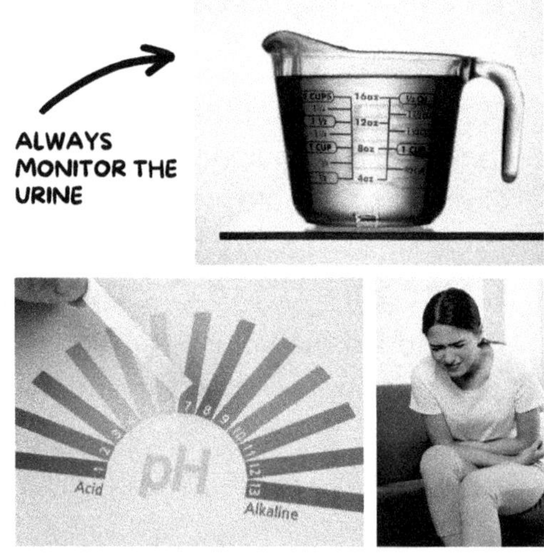

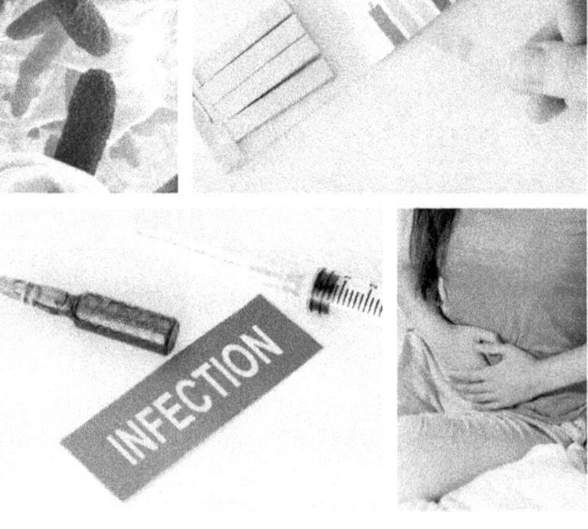

CHAPTER 8
PERSONAL HYGIENE AND DIGNITY

Personal Hygiene and Dignity

In this chapter, we will explore the importance of personal hygiene and dignity in catheter care. We'll discuss best practices for maintaining hygiene, techniques to ensure patient comfort and dignity, and strategies for addressing and preventing potential embarrassments. Additionally, we'll highlight the importance of hygiene around the catheter site and the specific considerations for men, including cleaning behind the foreskin to prevent complications like sepsis and split penis.

Importance of Personal Hygiene
Personal hygiene is paramount in catheter care to prevent infections, skin irritations, and other complications.

Sepsis

Sepsis is a life-threatening condition caused by the body's extreme response to an infection. It triggers widespread inflammation, leading to tissue damage, organ failure, and potentially death. Early recognition and treatment are crucial to improving outcomes and reducing the risk of severe complications.

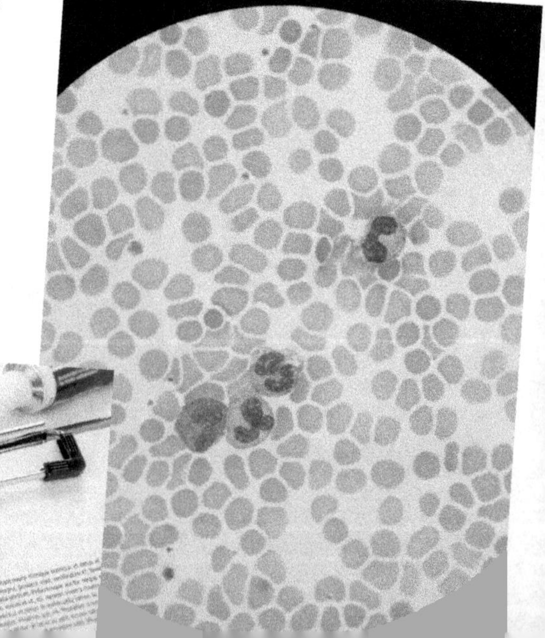

Importance of Personal Hygiene

Personal hygiene is paramount in catheter care to prevent infections, skin irritations, and other complications. Here are some best practices to ensure proper hygiene:

1. Periurethral Hygiene:
- Clean the periurethral area and catheter insertion site daily with mild soap and water.
- Gently pat the area dry after cleaning to prevent moisture build-up.

2. Hand Hygiene:
- Practice thorough hand hygiene before and after handling the catheter or drainage system to prevent contamination.
- Use soap and water or alcohol-based hand sanitizers to effectively clean hands.

3. Catheter Care:
- Ensure that the catheter and drainage system are kept clean and free from contamination.
- Regularly assess the catheter site for signs of redness, swelling, or irritation.

Techniques for Patient Comfort and Dignity

Maintaining patient comfort and dignity is essential in catheter care to promote trust and cooperation. Here are some techniques to ensure patient comfort and dignity:

Privacy:
- Provide privacy during catheter care procedures to respect the patient's dignity.
- Close curtains or doors and use drapes to maintain privacy during catheter insertion or catheter care tasks.

Communication:

- Communicate openly and respectfully with the patient about catheter care procedures.
- Encourage patients to express any concerns or preferences regarding their care.

Empowerment:

- Involve patients in their care decisions and empower them to participate in catheter management tasks to the best of their ability.
- Offer support and encouragement to boost patients' confidence and sense of control over their situation.

Addressing and Preventing Potential Embarrassments

Catheter care can sometimes lead to embarrassing situations for patients. Caregivers should be sensitive to these concerns and take steps to address and prevent potential embarrassments:

1. Anticipate Needs:

- Anticipate the patient's needs and provide assistance proactively to minimize embarrassment.
- Offer disposable pads or absorbent garments to manage leaks or accidents discreetly.

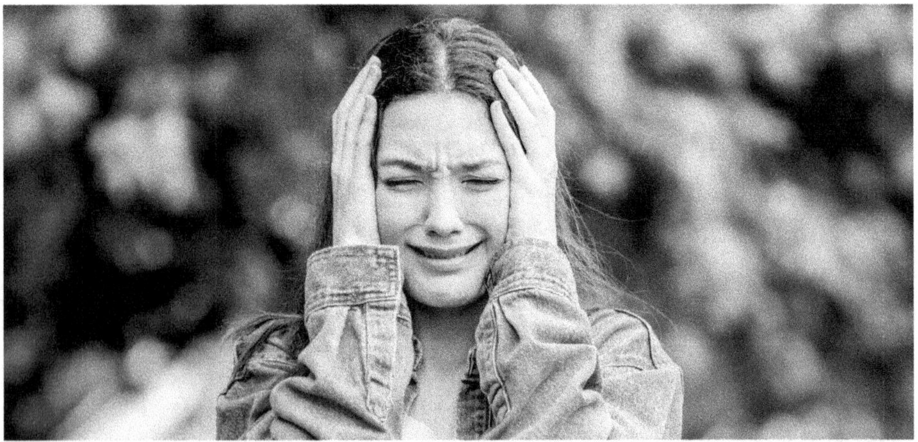

2. Use Discretion:

- Handle catheter care tasks with discretion and sensitivity, avoiding unnecessary exposure or discomfort for the patient.
- Use drapes or blankets to cover the patient during catheter insertion or catheter care procedures.

3. Provide Emotional Support:

- Offer emotional support and reassurance to patients who may feel embarrassed or vulnerable during catheter care.
- Validate their feelings and offer encouragement to help alleviate their concerns.

Special Considerations for Men

Men require additional hygiene considerations, particularly regarding cleaning behind the foreskin to prevent complications like sepsis and split penis. Caregivers should:

1. Foreskin Hygiene:

- Gently retract the foreskin and clean the area underneath with warm water and mild soap.
- Rinse thoroughly and dry the area to prevent moisture build-up and bacterial growth.

2. Education:

- Educate male patients and caregivers about the importance of foreskin hygiene and the potential risks of poor hygiene, such as infection and injury.

3. Monitoring:

- Monitor the catheter site and the area behind the foreskin regularly for signs of infection, inflammation, or other issues.
- Promptly report any abnormalities to healthcare providers for further evaluation and management.

Smegma

Smegma is a natural substance composed of shed skin cells, skin oils, and moisture. It accumulates in the genital area, particularly under the foreskin in males and around the clitoral hood in females. While smegma itself is not harmful, poor hygiene can lead to its buildup, which may cause irritation, inflammation, and an unpleasant odor. This environment can also foster bacterial growth, increasing the risk of infections such as balanitis in males and bacterial vaginosis or yeast infections in females. Regular cleaning is essential to prevent these issues and maintain genital health.

Conclusion

In conclusion, maintaining personal hygiene and dignity is essential in catheter care to ensure patient safety, comfort, and well-being. By following best practices for hygiene, techniques for patient comfort and dignity, and strategies for addressing and preventing potential embarrassments, caregivers can provide compassionate and respectful care to patients undergoing catheterization.

In the next chapter, we will discuss practical tips and strategies for effective catheter management, including maintaining accurate records and addressing common challenges in catheter care. With a comprehensive understanding of catheter care principles, caregivers can continue to uphold the highest standards of patient-centred care and promote positive outcomes for patients.

PERSONAL HYGIENE IS IMPORTANT

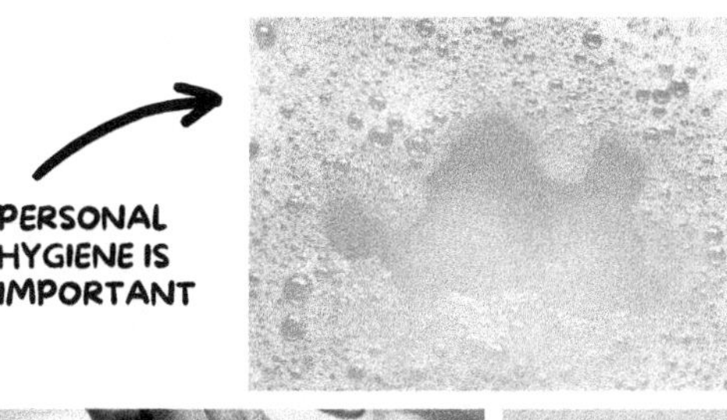

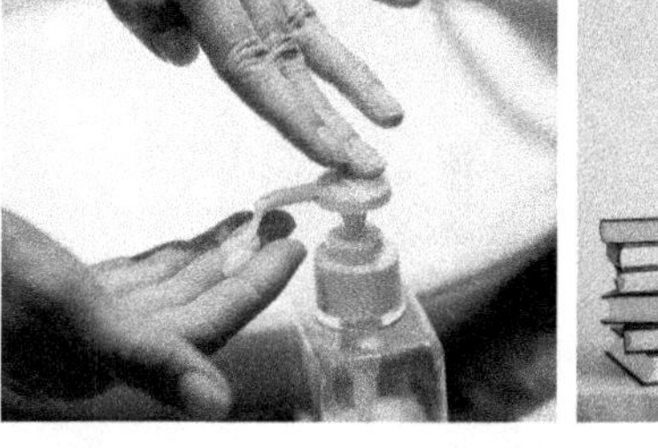

IT CAN PREVENT INFECTIONS

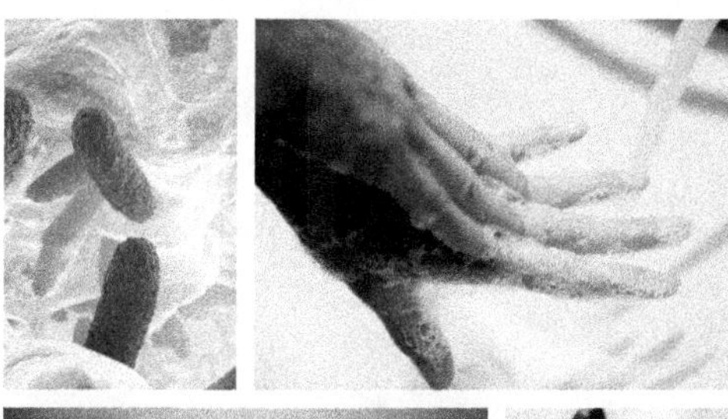

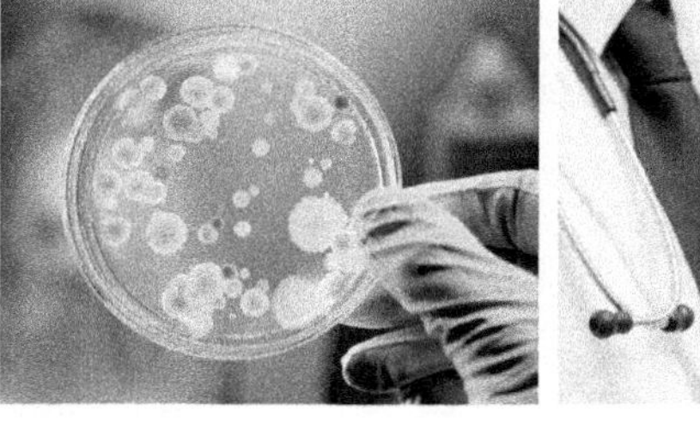

CHAPTER 9
HANDY TIPS AND WHY WE NEED TO KEEP A RECORD

Tips

Tips and Why We Need to Keep a Record

In this chapter, we will provide practical tips for carers on catheter care and discuss the importance of accurate record-keeping in ensuring the well-being of patients. Effective catheter management requires diligence, attention to detail, and proactive communication. By following handy tips and maintaining thorough records, carers can enhance the quality of care provided and promote positive outcomes for patients undergoing catheterisation.

Be Proactive

Being proactive in care, especially for catheter care, is essential to prevent complications and ensure patient well-being. Proactive measures include regular monitoring for signs of infection, smaintaining proper hygiene, and ensuring correct catheter placement and maintenance. These actions help minimize risks such as urinary tract infections, sepsis, and other complications. By anticipating potential issues and addressing them promptly, caregivers can significantly improve health outcomes, enhance patient comfort, and reduce hospital readmissions. Ultimately, proactive care fosters a safer, more effective healthcare environment, prioritizing patient safety and quality of life.

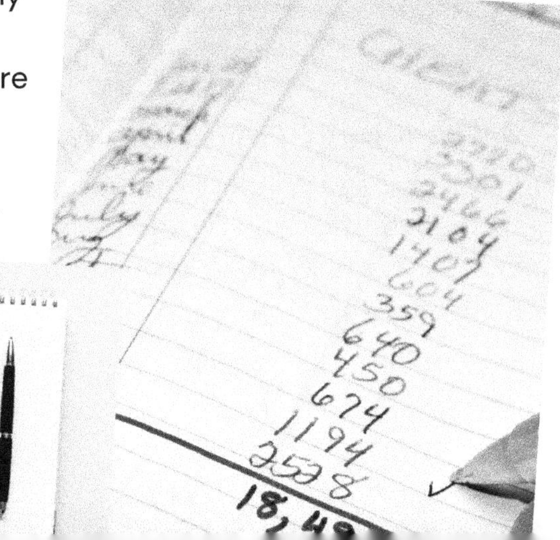

Practical Tips for Carers on Catheter Care

Caring for patients with catheters requires specialized knowledge and skills. Here are some practical tips for carers to ensure effective catheter management:

1. Proper Hygiene Practices:

- Emphasize the importance of hand hygiene before and after handling the catheter or drainage system to prevent infection.
- Clean the catheter insertion site regularly with mild soap and water and keep the surrounding area dry.

2. Secure Catheter Placement:

- Ensure that the catheter is securely taped or fastened to prevent accidental displacement.
- Monitor the catheter site for signs of irritation or skin breakdown and report any concerns to healthcare providers.

3. Monitor Urine Output:

- Measure and record urine output regularly to assess kidney function and fluid balance.
- Report any significant changes in urine output, such as sudden increases or decreases, to healthcare providers promptly.

4. Encourage Fluid Intake:

- Encourage patients to maintain adequate fluid intake to prevent dehydration and promote urinary flow.
- Monitor fluid intake and output to ensure proper hydration and kidney function.

5. Promote Comfort and Dignity:

- Respect the patient's privacy and dignity during catheter care procedures.
- Use drapes or blankets to maintain privacy during catheter insertion or catheter care tasks.

Importance of Accurate Record-Keeping

Accurate record-keeping is essential in catheter care to track patient progress, monitor for complications, and facilitate communication among healthcare providers. Here's why keeping detailed records is crucial:

1. Fluid Monitoring:

- Recording fluid intake and output helps assess kidney function, fluid balance, and the effectiveness of catheterization.
- Changes in urine output can indicate underlying medical issues or complications that require prompt intervention.

2. Documenting Changes and Complications:

- Recording changes in the patient's condition, such as fever, pain, or changes in urine characteristics, helps identify potential complications early.
- Documenting interventions and outcomes allows for continuity of care and ensures that all healthcare providers are informed of the patient's progress.

3. Communication and Collaboration:

- Detailed records facilitate communication and collaboration among members of the healthcare team, ensuring that everyone is aware of the patient's care plan and progress.
- Accurate documentation helps prevent errors, misunderstandings, and gaps in care that could compromise patient safety.

Documenting Changes, Complications, and Interventions

When documenting catheter care, carers should include the following information:

1. Catheter Care Procedures:
- Document details of catheter insertion, maintenance, and removal, including dates, times, and any observations or concerns.
- Record the type and size of catheter used, as well as any complications encountered during catheterization.

2. Fluid Intake and Output:
- Monitor and record fluid intake and output, including urine volume, colour, clarity, and odour.
- Note any changes in urine output or characteristics and report them promptly to healthcare providers.

3. Changes in Patient Condition:
- Document changes in the patient's condition, such as fever, pain, or signs of infection.
- Record any interventions performed, medications administered, and the patient's response to treatment.

4. Communication with Healthcare Providers:
- Document conversations and interactions with healthcare providers regarding the patient's care plan, concerns, and recommendations.
- Ensure that all communication is accurately recorded and easily accessible for future reference.

Conclusion

In conclusion, effective catheter management requires carers to follow practical tips for catheter care and maintain accurate records of patient progress and interventions. By adhering to proper hygiene practices, monitoring urine output, promoting comfort and dignity, and documenting changes and complications, carers can provide high-quality care and promote positive outcomes for patients undergoing catheterisation. Accurate record-keeping is essential for tracking fluid balance, monitoring for complications, and facilitating communication among members of the healthcare team. By documenting catheter care procedures, fluid intake and output, changes in patient condition, and communication with healthcare providers, carers can ensure that patients receive the best possible care and support throughout their catheterisation journey.

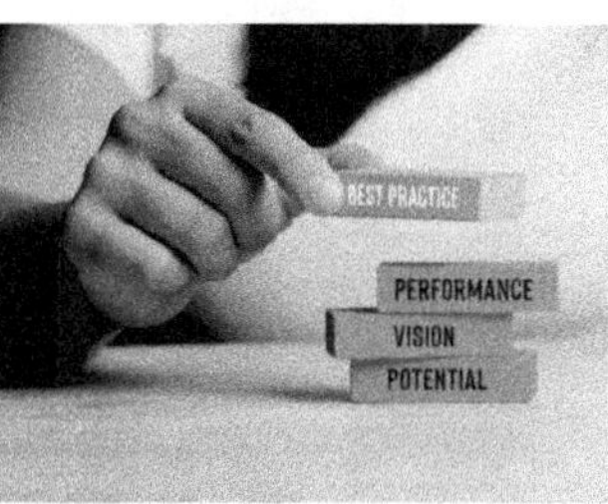

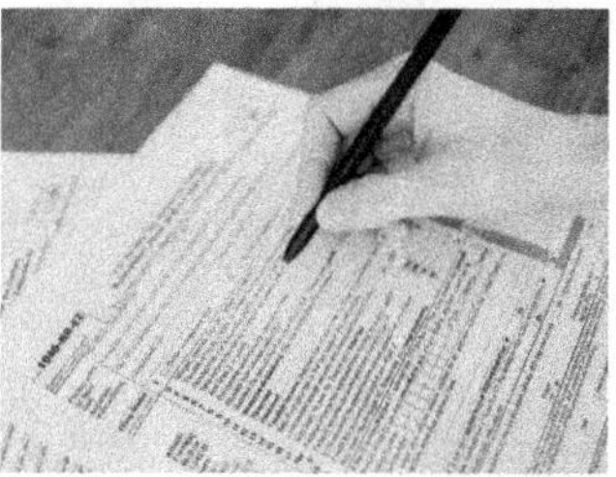

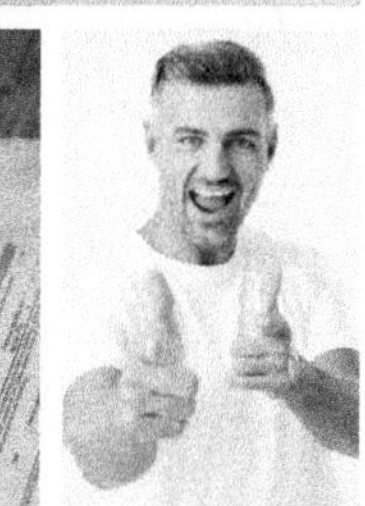

IT WILL REALLY ASSIST YOU!

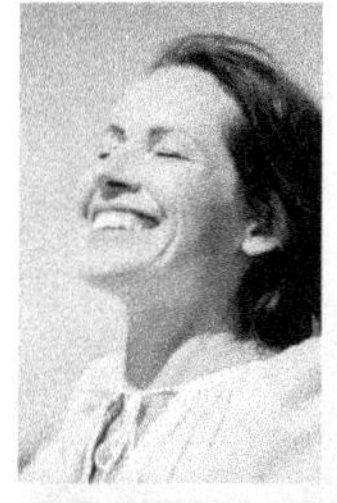

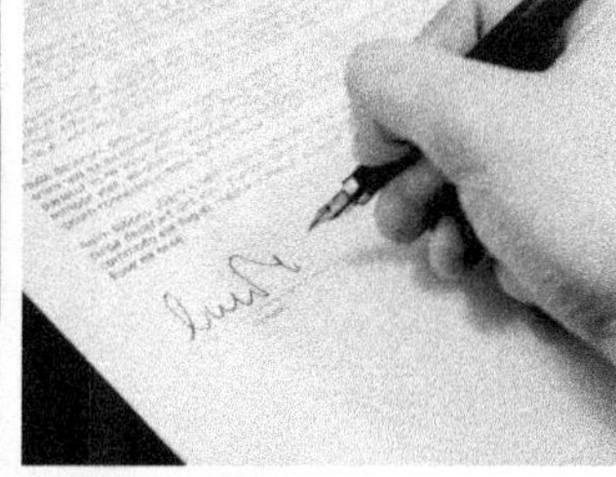

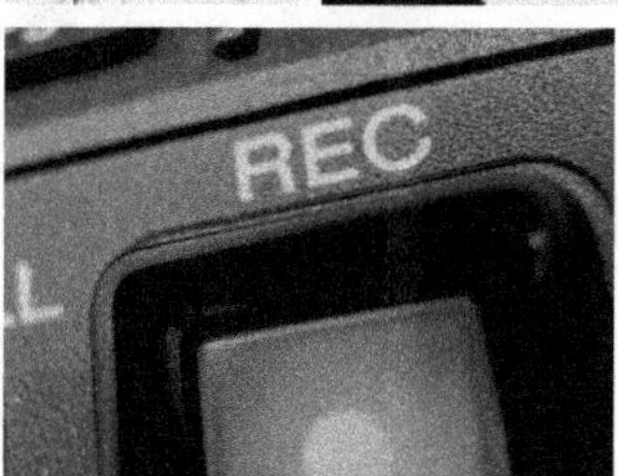

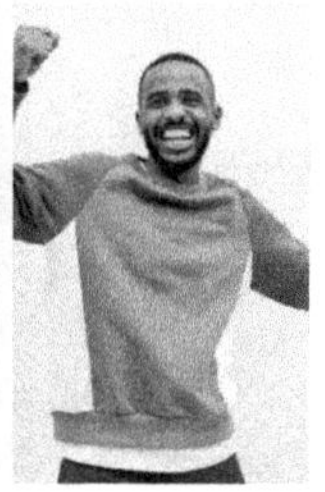

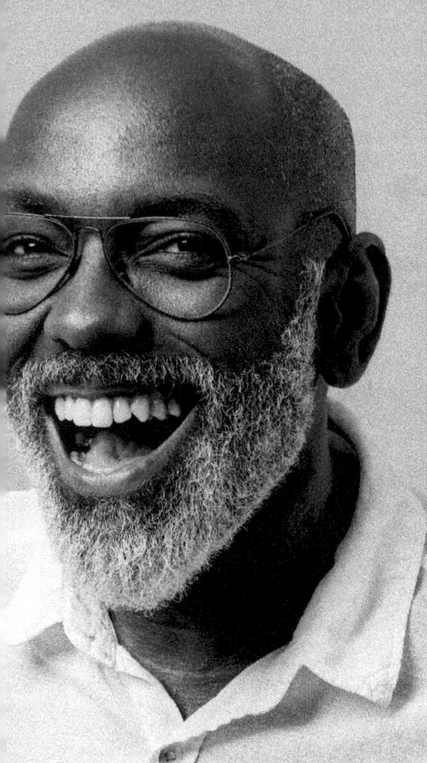

CHAPTER 10
SUMMARY

Let's Promote The Quality of Life

In this final chapter, we recap the key points discussed throughout this guide on catheter care. We emphasize the importance of proper catheter care, highlight the significance of maintaining patient dignity, and offer final thoughts on promoting quality of life for patients undergoing catheterisation.

Recap of Key Points

Throughout this guide, we have covered essential aspects of catheter care, including:

- Understanding what catheterisation is and its purposes, such as urinary drainage, diagnostic procedures, surgical use, medication administration, hydration, and nutrition.

- Exploring the history of catheterisation and milestones in its development, leading to modern catheter care techniques.

- Recognizing signs of infection or complications, ensuring proper catheter placement and maintenance, and monitoring urine output and quality.

- Implementing practical tips for carers on catheter care and emphasizing the importance of accurate record-keeping for tracking patient progress and interventions.

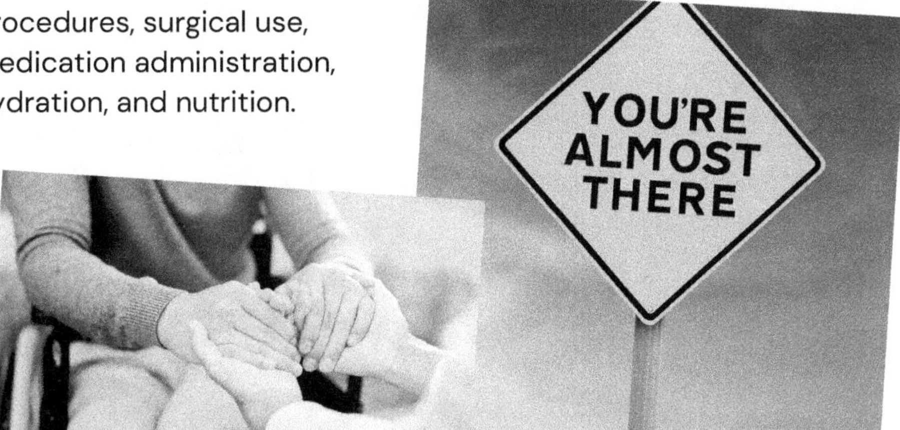

Importance of Proper Catheter Care

Proper catheter care is vital for ensuring patient safety, comfort, and well-being. By following best practices for hygiene, monitoring for complications, and maintaining accurate records, carers can minimize the risk of infection, promote optimal urinary function, and enhance the overall quality of care provided to patients.

Final Thoughts on Maintaining Patient Dignity and Quality of Life Maintaining patient dignity is paramount in catheter care. Carers should prioritize privacy, respect patient preferences, and empower patients to participate in their care decisions whenever possible. By promoting comfort, dignity, and autonomy, carers can help preserve the patient's sense of self-worth and quality of life throughout the catheterisation process.

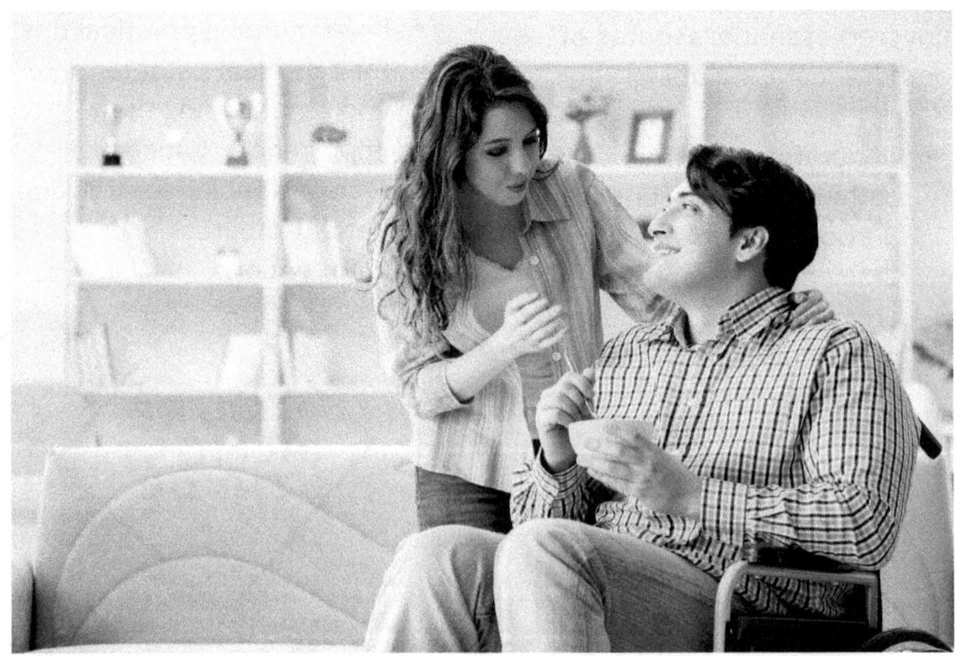

Conclusion

In conclusion, catheter care is a crucial aspect of healthcare that requires diligence, compassion, and attention to detail. By adhering to proper catheter care practices, carers can ensure optimal outcomes for patients undergoing catheterization, minimize the risk of complications, and uphold the principles of patient-centred care. With a commitment to maintaining patient dignity and promoting quality of life, carers can make a positive difference in the lives of those they care for, enhancing their overall well-being and comfort.

Thank you for reading this guide on catheter care. We hope that the information provided has been informative and valuable for your caregiving journey. If you have any further questions or concerns, please do not hesitate to seek guidance from healthcare professionals or other resources available to you.

THANKYOU FOR TAKING THE TIME TO READ THIS!

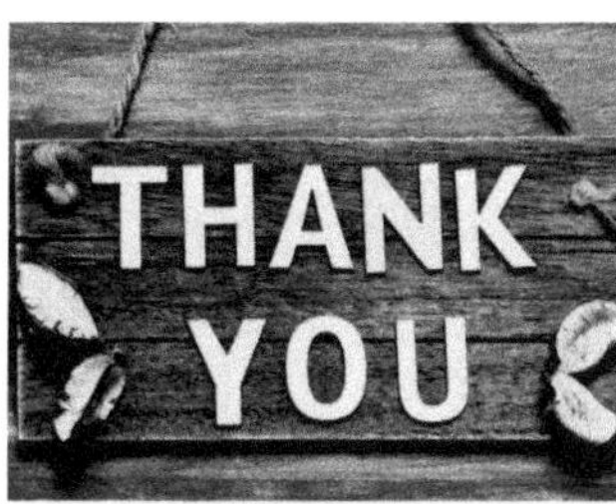

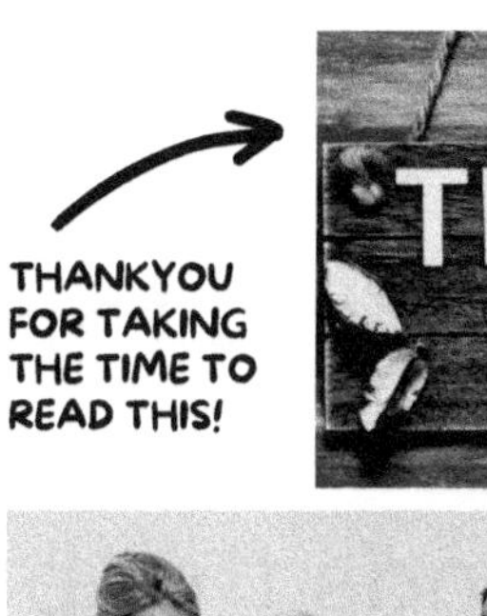

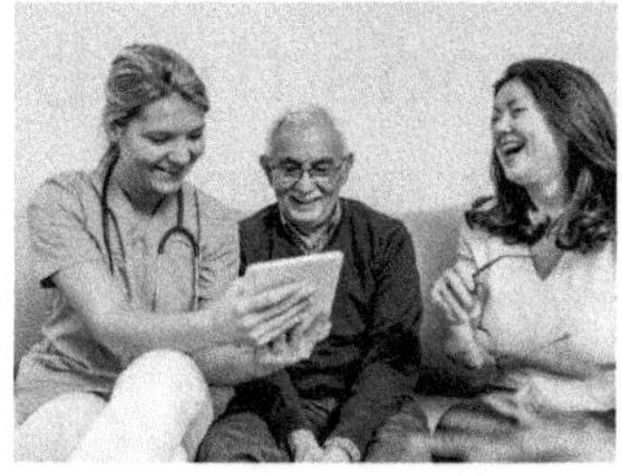

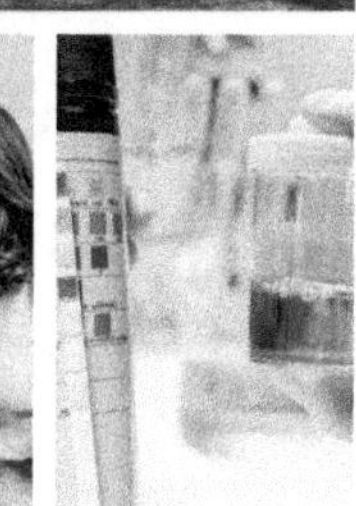

WE HOPE IT HELPS YOU!

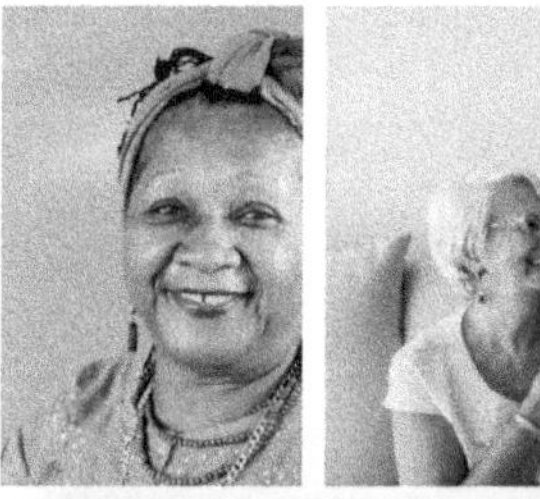

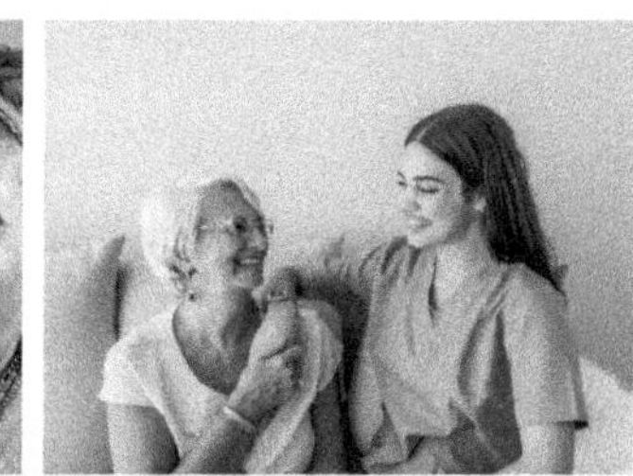

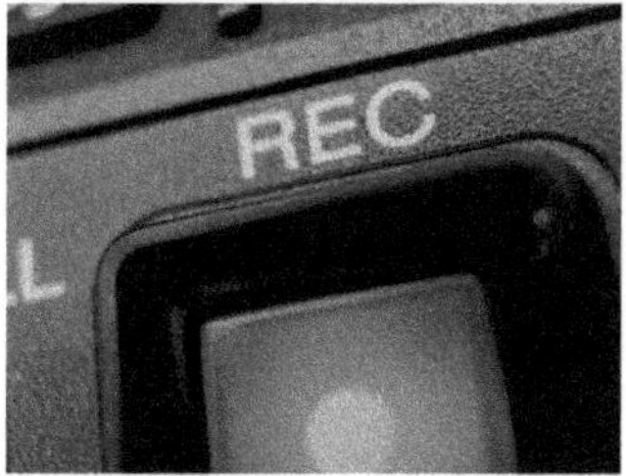

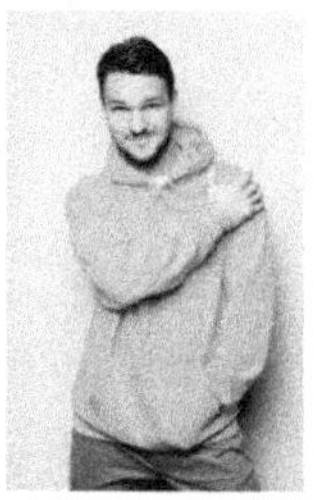

THE END

Here ends this book, but it could be the start of your journey. Keep looking forward but remember the past. Thankyou for reading!

ACKNOWLEDGEMENTS

I extend my heartfelt gratitude to all who have contributed to the creation of "I Need To Go To The Toilet." Firstly, I wish to express my appreciation to the individuals whose stories have inspired this work. Your courage and resilience have illuminated the pages of this book, and I am deeply honored to have had the opportunity to share your experiences.

To the photographers whose captivating images adorn these pages, sourced from copyright-free platforms such as Canvas, thank you for your artistry and generosity. Additionally, I am grateful for the additional photographs captured by myself, Roy Langstaffe, which have enriched the visual narrative of this book.

Furthermore, I wish to acknowledge that any person mentioned in this book has had their names altered to safeguard their privacy and protect their identity.

Lastly, to my family, friends, and colleagues who have provided unwavering support and encouragement throughout this endeavor, I am profoundly grateful. Your belief in me has been a constant source of strength, and I am indebted to each of you for your unwavering support.

With deepest appreciation,

ALSO BY THE SAME AUTHOR

ME, MYSELF AND THE OTHER ONE

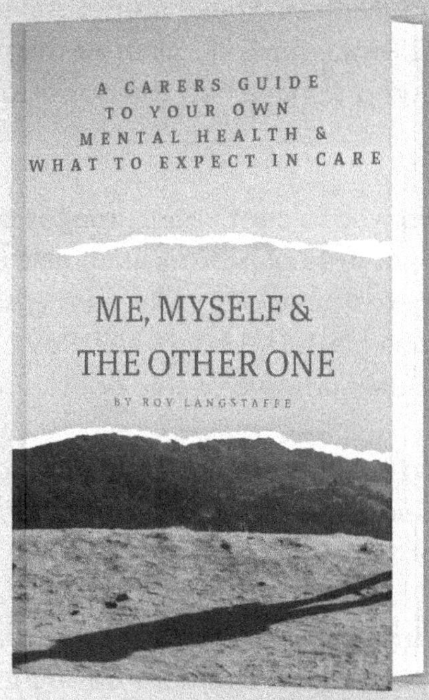

ROY LANGSTAFFE

ME, MYSELF AND THE OTHER ONE: A CAREGIVER'S GUIDE TO MENTAL HEALTH & WHAT TO EXPECT IN CARE IS ESSENTIAL FOR ALL CAREGIVERS, OFFERING PRACTICAL ADVICE, EMOTIONAL SUPPORT, AND INSPIRATION THROUGH TALES, QUOTES, AND POEMS. A TRUE COMPANION FOR YOUR CAREGIVING JOURNEY.

ALSO BY THE SAME AUTHOR

A DIFFERENT KIND OF NORMAL

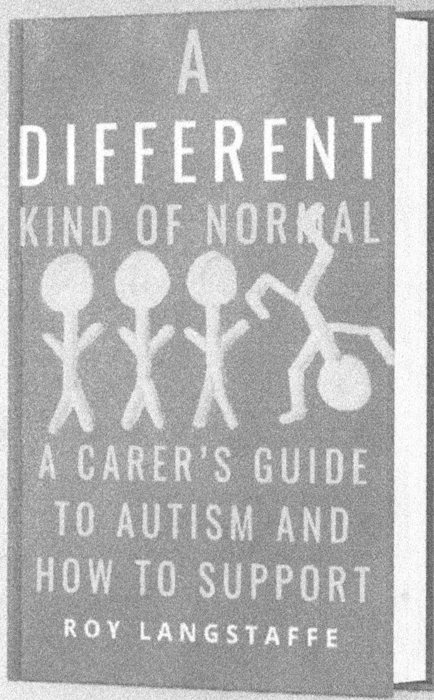

ROY LANGSTAFFE

A DIFFERENT KIND OF NORMAL: A CARER'S GUIDE TO AUTISM AND HOW TO SUPPORT IS ESSENTIAL FOR ALL CAREGIVERS, OFFERING PRACTICAL ADVICE, TIPS, AND INSPIRATION THROUGH INFORMATION AND REAL LIFE EXAMPLES OF HOW TO SUPPORT SOMEONE WITH AUTISM. IF YOU CARE, THIS IS ESSENTIAL READING!

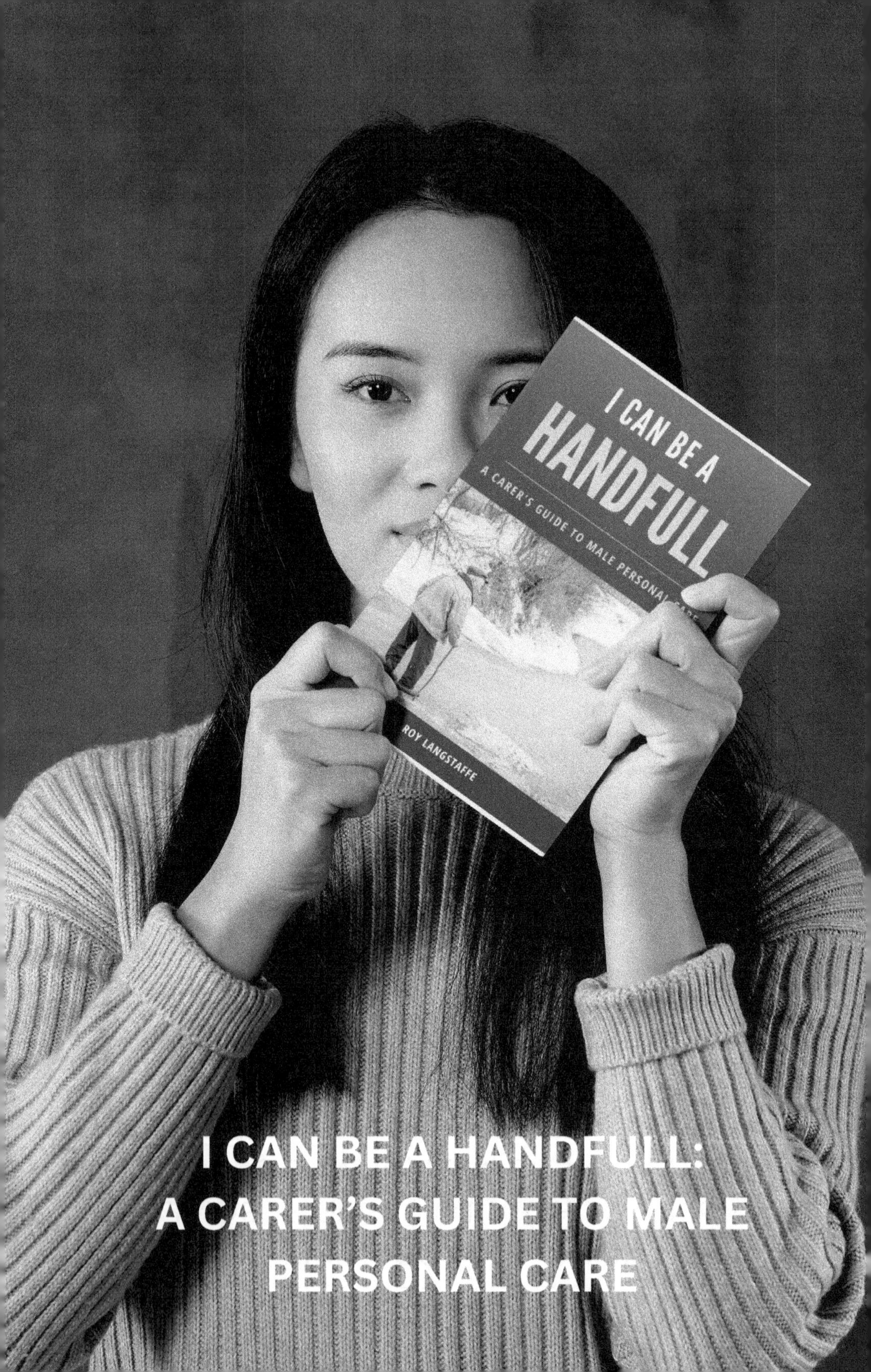
I CAN BE A
HANDFULL
A CARER'S GUIDE TO MALE PERSONAL CARE
ROY LANGSTAFFE
I CAN BE A HANDFULL:
A CARER'S GUIDE TO MALE
PERSONAL CARE

Disclaimer

© 2024 Roy Langstaffe. All rights reserved. No part of this publication, "I Need To Go To The Toilet," may be reproduced, distributed, or transmitted in any form or by any means, including photocopying, recording, or other electronic or mechanical methods, without the prior written permission of the publisher, except in the case of brief quotations embodied in critical reviews and certain other noncommercial uses permitted by copyright law.

The information contained in this book is for general informational purposes only. The author assumes no responsibility for errors or omissions in the contents of the book. The information is provided on an 'as is' basis with no guarantees of completeness, accuracy, usefulness, or timeliness.

This book is not intended to provide medical, legal, or financial advice. Readers are advised to seek the services of a qualified professional in these fields.

While the author has made every effort to ensure that the information in this book is correct, the author does not assume and hereby disclaims any liability to any party for any loss, damage, or disruption caused by errors or omissions, whether such errors or omissions result from negligence, accident, or any other cause.

This book may contain links to external websites that are not provided or maintained by or in any way affiliated with the author. Please note that the author does not guarantee the accuracy, relevance, timeliness, or completeness of any information on these external websites.

Photos provided by Canva are copyright-free. All other photos are by Roy Langstaffe.

www.ingramcontent.com/pod-product-compliance
Lightning Source LLC
Chambersburg PA
CBHW072338270726
48659CB00022B/1916